# Believe You Can & You Will: A Survivor's Guide To Health And Healing

Gail Keehn Dvoretz

Copyright © 2019 Gail Keehn Dvoretz

All rights reserved.

ISBN: 978-1-703-44324-0

## DEDICATION

For Janice Keehn

# CONTENTS

|  |  |  |
|---|---|---|
|  | Acknowledgments | i |
|  | Preface | iii |
| I. | **Rules Of Survival** | 1 |
| 1 | Let Go Of Unfortunate Beginnings | 2 |
| 2 | Obstacles Are There For A Reason | 9 |
| 3 | You're Allowed To Be Sad | 14 |
| 4 | Gail's Rules For Getting Through The Storms | 20 |
| 5 | Diabetes – Accept And Conquer | 25 |
| 6 | The Medi-Jector – Changing The Course Of My Disease | 28 |
| 7 | It Ain't Easy, But Make Food Your Friend | 31 |
| 8 | The FDA Is FOS | 37 |
| 9 | Work Hard – Play Hard | 41 |
| 10 | When Life Deals You A Bad Hand, Go Ahead And Play It | 44 |
| 11 | 2009 – Gluten Free Gail Is Born | 47 |
| 12 | It's Never Too Late | 50 |
| 13 | Breaking Up Is Hard To Do | 53 |
| II. | **Are You Ready To Detox? What's In Your Everyday Foods** | 61 |
| 14 | A2 Vs A1 Cows And The Benefits Of Raw Milk | 62 |
| 15 | BPA and BPAF – Don't Touch The Reciepts | 65 |
| 16 | Butter – The Real Deal | 69 |
| 17 | Canned Tomatoes – Not So Healthy | 72 |
| 18 | Carrageenan – A "Healthy" Additive? | 74 |

| 19 | Chemical Warfare Every Day | 77 |
| --- | --- | --- |
| 20 | Chocolate Exposed | 85 |
| 21 | Corn – The GMO Kind | 88 |
| 22 | Fish – Something's Fishy | 91 |
| 23 | Gluten Almost Killed Me – What Could It Be Doing To You? | 93 |
| 24 | Glyphosate – Be Afraid, Be Very Afraid | 97 |
| 25 | Heavy Metal – Not The Music, The Poison | 99 |
| 26 | It Ain't Honey, Honey | 102 |
| 27 | Nuts – A No No | 104 |
| 28 | Organic All The Way | 107 |
| 29 | Sourdough Bread – Crazy Healthy | 110 |
| 30 | Soy – So Confusing | 112 |
| 31 | Stevia – Not Worth The Risk | 115 |
| 32 | Sugar – Dangerously Sweet | 117 |
| 33 | Tin Foil (Isn't Anymore) | 120 |
| 34 | Wheat – Not The Way Grandma Remembers It | 123 |
| II. | **Are You Ready To Detox? Medical** | 126 |
| 35 | Cataracts Be Gone! | 127 |
| 36 | Statins – Not The Only Option | 130 |
| 37 | Thermography Vs Mammography | 133 |
| 38 | Vitamins – Here's The Scoop | 135 |
|  | Afterword | 138 |
|  | Shopping | 141 |
|  | Recipes | 152 |

# ACKNOWLEDGMENTS

There are several people I would like to acknowledge. They have seen me through thick and thin, inspired me, and in some cases, saved my life. The few mentioned here have really made a huge difference, but of course there are many others.

To my mother who turned me into a cold hard tough human being, which in the end saved my life.

To my father who failed as a parent but gave me a sense of humor to weather the storms I would eventually face.

To Jonathan, Brett and Charya, Francesca and her family - you all made my world better. Thank you for sharing your lives with me. You make it worth living!

To my sister Lannie who went on this horrible journey with me and stood by my side no matter how crazy my ideas were or what I wanted to do. You are the special person in my life who never criticized me or even got mad when I turned ugly. You are kind and loving to all who come your way. I learned to love again thanks to you. Please know that you are smart, beautiful, sincere, caring, and warm. You deserve the same from everyone in your life.

To Sammy, Meghan, and Alison - thank you for being part of our family. We look forward to more happy times together.

To Larry Eferstein, my loving and generous husband. They broke the mold when they made you. You saved my life every night for 20 years because my low blood sugars. You let me travel and help others while you held down the fort at home. You encouraged me to write this book so I could share my journey and my knowledge with others. You were the father my children never had and the parent I never had. Thank you for loving me and letting me finish my bucket list and not ever look back to say "I should have." You are special and kind, even though your childhood was no picnic either. You did all the right things as a husband, brother-in-law to my sister, and father to my children. My diabetes didn't scare you away. Instead, you promised that if I lost my vision, you would steer the bike and I could always pedal. You are my hero.

To my grandson Landon Totty, you will always hold a special place in my heart. You are so wonderful! You never forget to call or text. Thank you for including me in your childhood. Grandma Gail loves you.

To the only two doctors I trust: Dr. Ross Nochimson and Dr. Kenneth Tourgeman. Dr. Nochimson, you are an exemplary physician. You took care of my mother and now you take care of Lannie and me, and my sons, Jonathan and Brett. You are willing to listen to your patients, but you will also call and yell when someone is too stubborn to listen. Dr. Kenneth Tourgeman, I met you ten years ago and you actually knew that I was doing the right thing. You are also what a great doctor should be. I love you both and I want you to know that doctors like you are hard to find.

I would also like to thank my editor, and now friend, Patty Nolan of About the Words. She pushed and pulled me through this tough process. She made me aware of the value I was providing and encouraged me to see this book through. Patty put the pieces of my puzzle together, and if the dog ate my homework, she filled in the gaps. Without her this book would not have gotten done and I would have died with this important information inside of me. Thank you so very much Patty.

# PREFACE

I shouldn't be alive. There were many times in my life when I struggled with heartache, pain, and devastating illness. Against all odds, I made it through. I am 70 and healthy. My mission is to tell my story, but also to encourage people to take control of their health and their lives. I want people to own their choices. This book is packed with advice, guidance, and information, but it's not a quick fix. I won't tell you it's going to be easy. It's not. I became a human guinea pig so you don't have to, but my journey too is ongoing. I have to stay the course and continue to search for answers. I'm willing to do it. I'm willing to make sacrifices. I'm still climbing my stairway to health.

If you're not willing to dive in headfirst and do all the work, this book is still for you. Some health changes are better than none. But remember, full commitment is always better. You need to be open-minded. You need to <u>want</u> to change and get healthy. It is important to give your health 100% effort. Like I tell my friends and family, you can't be a little bit pregnant! It's the same with making a major change in life. You either do it or you don't. If you dabble, it will help, but it won't get the same results. My sister and I had to go full throttle so we could live. We had no choice. Maybe you're facing a similar health crisis and have no choice either. We did it, and so can you. Even if you're not, make this commitment and reap the rewards.

I've spoken at length to many friends and acquaintances over the years about what I did to save my own life. I've explained the major lifestyle changes it required including reading every label, cutting out certain ingredients completely, cooking my own meals, and rarely dining out. Most of them have chosen to ignore me or even ridicule me. My advice went in one ear and out the other. Now, years later, one by one those friends and acquaintances are getting sick. They are falling victim to the 21st century catalog of autoimmune diseases, from ALS to Scleroderma.

All autoimmune diseases are deadly – and if you live with regular flare-ups – maddening. The people I know and tried to help who are now plagued with these miserable maladies could have prevented them or kept them at bay by doing what I've done. But as we know, many live in "it isn't going to happen to me" denial. One by one they have all come back for help and in some situations all I can say is, "you can try to do what I did now, but I can't guarantee the same results." Of course it doesn't hurt to try. When does it become too late to live healthier lives? Never! It's never too late to give up unhealthy behaviors, (and those bagels), but the sooner the better.

With health declining in America, many turn to western medicine for healing. Sadly, the pills that are prescribed merely mask the core issues. These prescriptions may prolong life, but it's not always a healthy life. In many cases the medicine is doing more harm than good. I learned this the hard way as well, and I was determined to change what was going on in my life and health. The 39 prescription medications I was taking when I started healing my body were not fixing anything. They were masking what was truly going on. I had to make lifestyle choices that prevented my body from getting any sicker. I did the research. I educated myself. I made the sacrifices.

I truly hope that the information I share with you in this book will help you make better choices for yourself and your family. I hope you will take the advice to heart and not wait until it's too late. I hope you will take steps to eliminate the poisons and toxins hiding in your food and in your life. It's what I had to do, and it worked. I've done most of the heavy lifting so you don't have to. I've tried everything and isolated what works. I was motivated by a burning desire to get out of bed again and start dancing as fast as I could. I don't ever want to stop dancing and I don't want to die from anything but old age.

I've divided this book into two main parts. The first part is an abridged autobiography. I don't include it because I want to talk about my life. On the contrary, there are many episodes in my life that I would like to forget! I include this partial autobiography because I believe that whatever predisposition I had to be sick manifested and indeed exploded because of my life experiences. I am certain that my life and my illnesses are connected.

You may say that not everyone has had so many miserable life events, and therefore will most likely not get as sick as I did. That may be true. But I'd also argue that eventually, bad lifestyle choices catch up, whether your life has been charmed or cursed. Why take the risk and assume you'll skate by unscathed? Why not take control of your health? Your old age will thank you for it, believe me.

The second major part of this book I have called Are You Ready To Detox? It's no secret that Big Pharma, Monsanto, most doctors, and even the American Cancer Society don't really want us to get healthy. Healthy doesn't make people rich. There's no money in healthy. There's money in disease. Manufacturers of everything - from cosmetics, to carpets, to pills, to food - are conspiring to make us sick. Big corporations gamble with our health by using toxins and carcinogens in everything they mass-produce. They do NOT have our best interests in mind as they run their businesses. In the last decade there has definitely been an increase in awareness of their misdeeds, but I find that people still can't believe that the food and drug industries would purposely do harm. Well, I've got news for you. They have, they are, and they will continue to do so unless we take a stand. The final parts of the book are packed with recipes and resources to help you take back your health and your life.

Don't stick your head in the sand one day longer. Don't wait until you are too broken to be fixed. Read this book carefully and learn what to do to make informed and healthy choices. I did, and it has paid dividends. I chose, among other things, to follow a healthy diet made up of NO Gluten, NO Corn, NO GMOs, NO chemicals, NO heavy metals, NO plastics. Instead I consumed coconut kefir, butyrate, prebiotics, and some real vitamins without chemicals (or what I call "mystery ingredients"), as well as many other things that I detail in this book. Only then did I come back from the dead. I became "Comeback Gail." As I told my son during one of my darkest periods of illness, "I'm not ready to die. When the time comes, I want to die dancing." I hope you're ready to choose life and health too. If so, read on. Because if you believe you can, you will.

# PART I: RULES OF SURVIVAL

# 1
# LET GO OF UNFORTUNATE BEGINNINGS

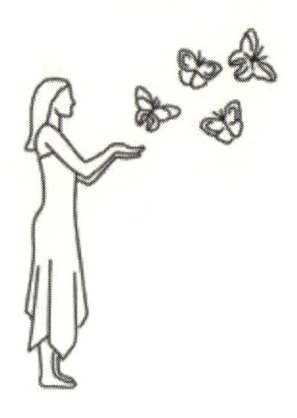

On June 18, 1949 I came into the world the way everyone else does but with one major difference. I was born to a mother who didn't want any more children - and should not have had any in the first place. From the day I was born I was in survival mode. My health was already compromised, and the party had just started.

My mother was an abuser. It didn't matter if you were a baby. My life as an infant started out with beatings and even though my entire family knew what she was doing, no one stopped her. Her sister, my Aunt Mimi, told me later that she thought about helping me but decided not to get involved. It's hard to understand that thought process. Let's not help the baby. Mind your own business and it will all go away. Bad people keep doing bad things, no one steps in, and the effects do not go away.

By the time I was six months old I was suffering from severe allergies and had pneumonia. My battle to survive had begun. I was given Aureomycin, an antibiotic prescribed in the 1940s. I should not have survived the pneumonia, but I did. However, my unhealthy gut started with that medical treatment and continued with the abuse I was getting from day one.

I grew up in a middle-class home on Long Island where my father worked in Manhattan and we didn't see him for much of the day. My father was the good guy and should have been the mother. I know now that my mother was bipolar, but at the time I just thought she was a mediocre parent occasionally, and an evil witch most of the time. When she was bad, she was horrid (as the poem goes).

I grew up with two sisters. My older sister Janice had her own issues, and sadly was similar to my mother in personality. She was absolutely gorgeous (as was my mother), but by age 14, she was a lost soul on her way to addiction. My younger sister Marlaine (we call her Lannie – pronounced Lay-knee) was seven years younger than me and I was very protective of her. I took it upon myself from a very early age to shield her from any physical abuse at the hands of my mother and Janice. I succeeded to a certain extent, but I couldn't protect her completely from our toxic environment and she too became sickly. While Janice turned to drugs, I turned to food for comfort. I cried all the way through elementary school as the kids tormented me and called me Gail the Whale. From a very early age, I believed myself to be short, fat, and stupid. Those were the messages I was getting from my mother and other bullies, and I believed them.

By the time I was 13 in 1962, my parents' marriage was on the rocks. My dad couldn't do anything right in my mother's eyes, and he finally stopped trying. We found out later that my mother had been having an affair. Eventually her paramour, Carl, would move into our home and become my stepfather.

I remember one particular event in my "sunny" childhood when my mother started beating me up in the kitchen over a smudge of dirt on her stove. By this age, I had already built a wall of protection around myself and was hardened to her madness, but my father had reached his breaking point. He threw the breakfast plates against the kitchen wall and said to her, "here's something for you to scream about. Feel free to act like a lunatic." He took my hand and walked out the door. We drove to my grandmother's house where he left me to figure out what he should do about this untenable situation. He knew he wouldn't be successful fighting for custody in court, and he wouldn't get any support from her family. After a week at my grandmother's, he came to pick me up and explained that he was leaving. He didn't know what else to do and he didn't know what to do about us. I told him to take care of himself and come back for us when he could. I promised I would take care of Lannie and we would both survive. The battle that was my life got worse that day. I was left in the hands of an increasingly crazy human being. My health was already an issue and with the life I was living, it was only a matter of time before I got really sick.

I went home after talking to my father that day and my mother didn't come near me for a month. She was preoccupied with the new man in her life. But one day, when I stood up for Lannie (age six) as she was being screamed at, the beatings began again. But I was a different person. I was no longer afraid for my life. She didn't have that power over me anymore. I had already gotten hard inside and I stopped caring what she did to me. She wanted me to fear her. Instead I just went cold. When she started to hit me I would stand up and smile in her face. I knew that drove her nuts because she would tell me to wipe that smile off my face. I didn't. I refused to cry and make her happy. I learned that tears didn't help. Being tough was the only thing that could get me through the day.

My school years were horrible as well. I was a very shy and quiet little girl and I had nothing to say for a very long time. As I continued to fail in school and struggled to read, my mother had to help me with my homework. This annoyed her and she became more aggressive and added "lazy" and "a procrastinator" to the litany of insults she hurled at me. I laugh now thinking back on all I have done in my life to become successful. Procrastinator was the last word that should have ever been used to describe me. Fear was always in my heart and that is why I procrastinated as a child. Fear of failing. Fear of beatings. Fear of insults. Fear was my constant companion. Amazingly, I did have one outlet that brought me great joy.

At the age of ten, three years before my dad left the family, I started sneaking over to my friend Marie's house to play her piano. I had never taken a lesson. I just knew how to play by ear. One of my other friends had an organ and when I tried that, I decided I liked it better because it was easier to push down the keys. I began to go to her house daily so I could play the organ. She couldn't believe how well I played without lessons. She herself was taking lessons and could barely figure it out. After a while I decided to make a bet with my dad. If I could play the organ would he get me one? He looked up laughing and said, "sure honey, if you can play it, I'll buy you one." That was the first time I prepared a written contract with signatures. I told him to pick the song and as long as I could sing it, I could play it on a keyboard. It took me two months of practice and in those two months I learned as much as I could about the Hammond Organ. Finally the moment of truth arrived.

Together we walked over to my friend's house and as Yankee Doodle Dandy played on TV, I sat down at the very big keyboard and played the entire show music and sang the songs as well. When I finished, I turned around and saw shock on my father's face. Up until then I had seemed like a timid and very dull little girl and out of nowhere emerged a musician who had never taken a music class in her life. Something sparked in me that day. I realized I wasn't stupid, just different. I may not have been beautiful and smart like Janice or dainty and cute like Lannie, but I was musically gifted and had found something I loved to do. A whole new world opened up me…I was doing something that no one else I knew could do. I could sit down at a musical instrument, turn on a record, and just play along. My dad kept his promise and bought me an organ. I would play only for my father or at night in secret. I refused to play for my mother because she said I was no good at it. She really never knew how well I could play, and she didn't really care. Instead she would scream out, "how can you remember the words to the songs and the keys on that stupid thing you play, and not be able to spell or read a damn fucking thing?" Yes, her language was chilling, especially to a child.

When my dad finally moved out, I knew I was in trouble. My mother went to work so I was safe during the day but at night things turned ugly. My older sister Janice and my mom had become a tag team. If one didn't get me, the other one did. I became their punching bag both emotionally and physically. Janice called me Cinderella because I had to cook, clean, and take care of Lannie while attending school. Janice refused to help out, so I had to do it all. She would beat me up as well. She had learned how to be an abuser from my mother. Music and the keyboard were my only escape. No one could touch me. My mother became increasingly upset that I refused to play the organ for her, so its removal became her new favorite threat. She demanded that I play and I continued to refuse. What she didn't know was that I cut school every day to come home and play. I even bought special plug-in headphones and I was up playing at night while everyone slept.

In an effort to humiliate me and prove how bad I was at playing the organ, when I was 15 my mother went behind my back and got me an audition at the Juilliard School of Music in Manhattan. I didn't have a clue what Juilliard was and it never dawned on me to ask how she got the interview. I know now that she couldn't believe how gifted I was, especially without a single lesson or a sheet of music. My fingers and feet would just fly naturally. That organ would take me away. I became someone other than short, fat, stupid, ugly Gail.

On the day of my audition, Jekyl had left the building and Hyde was in her place. It had been a fairly peaceful morning, but the calm did not last. Crazy lady was back in action and the yelling and screaming began over some pants lying on the floor in my bedroom. We all had to have perfect rooms every day. Pants on the floor were not allowed.

Despite the joyous occasion and unbelievable opportunity, my smile faded as we drove into Manhattan. Not one word was spoken between us. Gail was gone and in her place was the stone I had turned into. My mother's nasty streak would always rear its ugly head unexpectedly and that was never going to change. I could never let my guard down, and never let her fool me into thinking any day was going to be a good day.

The audition took place in St. Patrick's Cathedral where they had a huge organ. As soon as I saw it, I remember thinking how wonderful it would be to just sit and play that instrument! A very nice man introduced himself and we talked a little bit about how I started in music and when we were done he asked if I wanted to try the big organ with those long pipes going all the way up to the ceiling. I was in awe of the size of it, but not scared. I just wanted a chance to play. My mother sat silently watching me talk to this very nice man and as he smiled at me, I walked up to the organ, sat down, and gently ran my fingers across the keys. I was in love for the first time and it wasn't with a boy - it was with a musical instrument.

He told me to play whatever I wanted to and I could hear my mother blurting out that I never practiced. I laughed inside. Boy was she in for a shock. All I did was practice. I just made sure she wasn't around to see it. When I cut school I was at the keyboard. When I couldn't sleep at night I was at the keyboard. I was at the keyboard whenever she was gone and as far as I was concerned even though she sat right in front of me, she had been gone for years.

I chose Rhapsody in Blue and off I went into my own world. I heard nothing except the music. I had learned the entire song by listening to a record. It was a long song and I loved playing it. When I was done I looked up and saw my mother crying. The man asked her if she knew I could play like that. Sadly her answer was no and when she looked at me, for the first time I saw respect. However, at that point, it was too late. I no longer cared about how she felt or what she thought. I believe this is how health begins to decline. The connection between childhood abuse and chronic illness, in my view, is undeniable. I was abused, I was hardened, and I was going to face a lifetime of illness. Ironically, the same abuse that made me sick, in a twisted way prepared me for what I would face down the road.

When I completed the song, the man asked if I could sing and I said yes, but I was much more shy about singing in front of anyone other than Lannie. I took a deep breath and sang a Barbra Streisand song. He asked if I could dance and I told him I had taken tap many years ago and didn't know if I could dance anymore. Looking back on that remark I laugh because now, at 70 years of age, I dance five days a week. I live to dance and on Christmas Eve 2017 I got certified as a ZUMBA® instructor.

Once the audition was over he went and talked to my mother. I had not heard of the Juilliard School of Music so it was no big deal to me. I was never told what I was really getting out of that audition. I only knew that I did it to show my mom that I wasn't stupid, fat, or ugly. I could learn to do something and I could do it well. Again during the ride home I didn't speak to her. Instead I stared out the window planning my next move. I was admitted to Julliard, but I didn't attend.

All the hurt and anger I kept bottled up continued to tear away at my insides. I wonder, even if I had known that all that stuff was going make me sick could I have turned it around? If I had been a happy child, would the outcome have been different? Maybe. I think on some level, I became successful because I was determined to "show that witch." Should I thank her for instilling that drive in me, or would I still have it without my childhood of fear and terror?

After my parents' divorce, my father moved to Puerto Rico to develop properties. He wasn't around to help me but I managed to stay alive and somewhat protect Lannie. It wasn't easy but I did it. Of course my mother was very jealous and upset that I maintained a relationship with my father through the mail. When he came to New York for a visit, I lied to her and managed to see him. It was always a bone of contention with her.

When I turned 16 things escalated again. She continued her abuse, despite the fact that for years I had refused to show her any emotion at all. It all came to a head one night when I had been using her phone to talk to my dad. She said if I wanted to talk to him on the phone I should get my own phone. The next day I went out and got a job at the local pizza restaurant in Green Acres, New York. After my first paycheck, I bought my own phone and had it installed. When she came home I was on *my* phone with *my* father in *my* bedroom. She asked what I was doing and I told her. An insane look came over her. She pulled the phone out of the wall and told me I could not have a phone in her house and began to beat me with the handle. This was finally my breaking point. I really don't know what happened next but Gail was gone and another crazy young woman emerged. I turned around and with all my 5'2" strength hit my 5'10" lunatic mother in the face and knocked her to the floor. "Party over bitch," I thought to myself as I hit her. I could have killed my own mother that night. When she started to get up I grabbed a pair of scissors and said, "mom, don't get up because if you do I will have to kill you. Stay on the floor and I will get what I need and leave." She must have known I meant business because she did not get up as I gathered up bare essentials to make my escape. At that moment I didn't give a thought to my younger sister. I just had to leave in order to survive. I thought about going to Puerto Rico to live with my dad but I had no idea how to get to him. My Plan B was moving into my girlfriend's house but our parents knew each other so that was a bad Plan B. I ran out the door that night in a snowstorm and hitched by myself into Manhattan.

At the age of 16 I lived on the streets with the homeless for about two months eating out of garbage cans to survive. As grim as it might seem, those months were not so bad. I was free from the wicked witch. I didn't have to finish all the food on my plate. I didn't have to cook and shop. I didn't have to clean an entire house and I wasn't being beaten.

Living on the streets of Manhattan was actually a learning experience. I learned that the "bums," mostly homeless vets, were nicer to me than my own mother. I learned to steal from grocery stores for food. I learned that I didn't really need a bedroom to feel safe. All I needed were my wits to protect me. Living on the street with food not guaranteed taught me control. I had to plan my meals around what I could steal and what I could take from a garbage can. I lost 20 pounds in those two months and I was no longer Gail the Whale. I left home fat, quiet, and shy and returned a much stronger (and thinner) person. I decided then that I would never rely on anyone. I was going to make it on my own. I never looked back

# 2

# OBSTACLES ARE THERE FOR A REASON

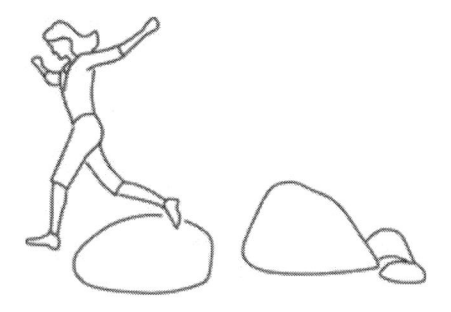

Living alone on the streets of Manhattan when I was not really a street kid took a turn for the worse after those two months. I needed and wanted a shower. I longed for food that was cooked that I didn't have to steal and I needed a job. What I really wanted was a normal home and family, but that was not in my cards. I was on my own and my brain had started to accept what I had done. I had nowhere to go and no way of letting anyone know where I was. School was becoming a thing of the past. The boy I was dating, Barry, didn't even know where I had gone. I decided that the best thing I could do was go back to my hometown of Elmont, get in touch with Barry and my best girlfriend Charlene, and see where that would lead. I also needed to go into school and let them know what was happening in my life. I had already visited the school psychologist earlier that year and he had warned me to get out before my mother killed me, (or I killed her). He was an intuitive man. I had followed his advice and ran, but now I needed to go back.

Thankfully when I got back to school and explained my situation, I was given permission to find a place to live and get back to school full-time. I got my job back at the Green Acres Mall pizza place and found a place to live. Barry's parents, after hearing my story, took me in and gave me the upstairs bedroom. They were the kind of parents everyone should have. They were warm, loving, and supportive. From this family I learned how good parents behaved. I started picking up books and began to read and study. My reading level was never going to be college level, or so I thought, but at least I was reading. I had always had trouble in school, a direct result of being told I was stupid by my mother, and struggled to pass any class that didn't involve art or music. Barry and his parents helped me study and life became wonderful because I was now reading. More proof that I wasn't stupid. When I had trouble with homework, Barry and his parents helped me lovingly – it was unbelievable.

I had people who cared, a boyfriend who helped me study, and a job that provided pocket money. Barry's parents would not take money from me for room and board so I began to learn about saving. I opened up my very first bank account and put money away for a rainy day. I finished 11th grade in 1966 living in Barry's family home and finally thriving. I began an exercise program to lose the baby fat I had left after my initial "street life" weight loss. To this day I exercise no matter how I feel or what I have going on in my day. Exercise is a must just like breathing. No more Gail the Whale. I wasn't thin by any means, but I was no longer 5'2" and 180 pounds. My life was good, and things were turning around. I had not spoken to my mother in three months, which was fine, but I hadn't spoken to Lannie either, and that bothered me.

Against my better judgment, I began to initiate contact with my mother so I could see my sister. When I did, she immediately told me she was going to sell my organ because I didn't live there and I no longer needed it. That wasn't what I wanted to hear. She then said if I moved back home I could keep it. She knew my plan was to get an apartment after graduation and she knew I wanted to take my organ with me. I stupidly believed her and moved home thinking things had changed.

For a few months she was tolerable but it didn't last long. She sold my organ out from under my nose. She couldn't help herself. She had to be nasty. I now know how sick she really was, bipolar and angry all the time. She had learned those behaviors from her mother and brother who were also abusive. She left home at 16 and married my father to escape. Her life wasn't pretty and she was mentally ill, so she became a monster. But that didn't help me cope at the time. Her behavior set my sisters and I up for major issues, both medically and emotionally. Janice was messed up and used drugs to numb her pain. I stopped my pain first by eating, and then by fighting back and fleeing. Lannie just retreated into herself. Her sweet, gentle, kind, and loving nature made her a target for victimhood. She lost her will to fight. She has been sickly a good deal of her life and continues to be so. She doesn't deserve the kind of life she now has. She lives with a mean nasty drunk. She married her mother, father, and drug addicted sister all rolled up into one. We seek out the people we think we deserve in life, based on the lessons of our childhood. If our childhood was bad, that equals terrible relationships until we get professional help and break the cycle. Lannie chooses to live with these ghosts of her past. A 12-step program has helped me deal with my demons and I still struggle.

I survived at my mom and stepfather Carl's until my high school graduation in June of 1967, which I did not attend because I was packing to get out of town. I boarded a plane to Puerto Rico to find my dad. As that plane took off, I smiled. I was finally free of her. I did feel the pain of leaving Lannie, but I was no good to her until I went out into the world to make a life for myself. Then I could go back for Lannie, which is exactly what I did.

I really didn't expect much from my father in the way of financial support but I knew that I would get emotional support and that was all I needed at that time. That combined with (and in contrast to) the anger and hatred toward my mother is what drove me to press on no matter what. I lived on that anger and it fueled all motivation. It probably also made my body a ticking disease time bomb, but it was all I had. I never spoke about my mother and the abuse for many years afterwards except to my father, who had lived it as well. I have since made peace with her and with all she put me through. When she was very old she apologized to me in her own way. I could have really let her have it, but I didn't. She was at the end of her life and by that time I had learned enough to know that she had also grown up in a sick dysfunctional household. It was all she knew. What good would it have done for me to destroy an old lady who knew she had behaved horribly and felt badly about it? I accepted her apology and I'm really glad I did. I was proud of myself for the way I handled it all. But that apology came many years after my high school graduation.

When I got to Puerto Rico in the summer of 1967, it didn't take me long to find my father. People in town knew who he was and where he would be later that day. I sat and waited at an Old San Juan hotel watching the people go by and decided that I should get a job there. It looked like a happy place to be. I just didn't know what to do yet and I didn't speak any Spanish. I set my sights on learning the language and doing something to make some money.

When my father showed up, the smile on his face let me know that I had made the right decision. Those open arms and the big hug I got were all I needed. We sat down and talked for hours. I opened up about everything: my life on the streets, Barry's parents taking me in, going back home, and the same torture continuing. I told him how mom had sold my organ and how she had showed me the letter the new owner had written to her about how happy she was playing it. Saying it out loud made it seem even worse. He asked if I wanted another one and I said no. I refused to play ever again. I had left that Gail behind.

I spent two years in Puerto Rico living with my father. I sang in a band and made enough money to live and even save a bit. My father had an apartment in San Juan and I immersed myself in my new life. I learned Spanish, rode a motorcycle throughout the rainforest, sang in a band, and casually dated some very nice local men.

This all came to an abrupt end when my girlfriend Charlene came to visit. We spent three weeks together and she suggested that I come home and make amends with my mom. The time was right for me to go back home and get some real direction, but not the right time to make amends with the wicked witch. I had had enough of Puerto Rico and didn't see a future singing at a San Juan hotel club. So despite my dad's protests, I went back home with Charlene and got an apartment.

I found a job on an assembly line at Garrard Turntables on Long Island. Music always seems to be in my life. After awhile there, I decided that college, instead of factory work, might be a good idea. Charlene thought I had lost my mind. I hadn't taken any college prep classes. I didn't start to read with any ease until the 11th grade, and only then because Barry's mom took me to Hofstra University to get tested to see if I was slow. She didn't think I was but I wasn't convinced yet. That's how much damage my mother had inflicted. The truth was the opposite. I was just a severely abused child who was actually really smart.

I applied to Nassau Community College in Garden City, NY, and was initially rejected for admission to the day program, which didn't really surprise me. I was used to adversity and I asked about options. I wanted this badly. I made an appointment with an advisor and explained why I had not taken any college prep classes and why I hadn't studied anything except art and cooking. She said I had an option and I immediately perked up. I love options. Life is always about Plan B. If you're not open to Plan B, you're in trouble. She said I could take nighttime entrance classes and if I passed those I could move to daytime classes and matriculate to a degree program. That was all I needed to hear.

I started with art classes, my second love, and began to pass bonafide college classes, including English and math, for the first time in my life. I then matriculated to a degree program. I began in the arts and somewhere along the way I moved to teaching art to disabled and mentally challenged kids. I could relate to them. I was on my way to making a career helping kids like myself - I just didn't know it yet. I found out in those years that I loved to learn just about anything - except biology. I passed out while dissecting a fetal pig and they moved me to a physics class. I may have been abused but my empathy was intact and I was a hopeless animal lover. Physics turned out to be the class from hell, but I made a Plan B and became friends with the teacher. I can now say "thank you Dr. Peterson," because without him I couldn't have passed that class and my dream of any kind of degree would have gone up in smoke. Two years later I was getting my AA degree in Art from Nassau Community College and I was ready to apply to a four-year school to continue my education.

By this time, I had moved in with another boyfriend and his family. He was also a wonderful human being. He was heading off to Pittsburgh in the fall for medical school so I decided to go with him. I applied to the University of Pittsburgh but they turned me down. I knew I didn't want to go there so I wasn't upset. Instead I applied to Duquesne University. I knew they had one of the best education programs in the United States. What I didn't know was that I, (a nice Jewish girl from Long Island), had applied to a Catholic college with Jesuit priests as professors. I applied again and they too said no, but I decided I wasn't going to let that be the final answer.

I felt compelled to make the eight-hour drive through the mountains alone to Pittsburgh to see the head of admissions at Duquesne. I was going to fight my way into that college. No one fights their way into a top tier university, do they? Well I did. I needed a chance to show that I was worthy. I needed someone to believe in me. As miserable as periods in my life have been, I have always been blessed with the right people put in my path at the right time. I found that person in the Dean of Admissions at Duquesne.

I got to the college at 9:00 a.m. and went to the office. I had been taking summer classes in Spanish, algebra, and science to get my average up. I was studying like crazy. I had very little money and always traveled with my own food. I waited through lunch and asked if I could study in the office while everyone else with money went to lunch. They said I could sit in study hall or in the cafeteria. I knew I needed a study hall so I went there and quietly ate my lunch and studied.

I fell in love with Duquesne University that day. I talked my way in by making an agreement with the Dean. I had to maintain a "B" average the first semester and once I did that I became a full-time matriculating student. I graduated from Duquesne with a degree in Special and Elementary Education. This was the early 1970s and special education was rarely taught as a specific education discipline. Duquesne had one of the only programs in the country that certified its teachers in every area of special education. It was a valuable degree that would serve me well later in life, give me a rewarding career, and eventually lead me to my current husband, Larry, with whom I've been for 30 years.

While my academic life was flourishing, my relationship with the man I had moved to Pittsburgh for and with did not last. I wasn't ready to be in a normal healthy loving relationship at the time. He was a good man and is now a very successful physician, but I just couldn't be the woman he wanted me to be. I had way too much work to do on myself. Despite my successes, I was still damaged goods. My ability to sustain a healthy loving relationship with a man would come years down the road with Larry.

# 3

## YOU'RE ALLOWED TO BE SAD

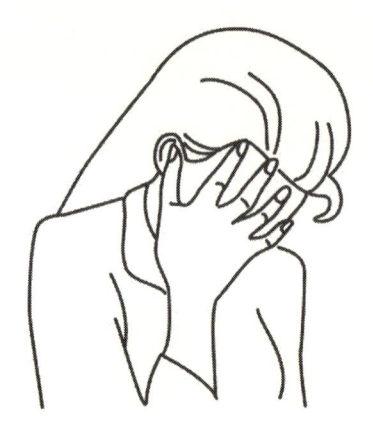

When I got back to New York in 1973 after finishing at Duquesne I moved in with my older sister Janice. Yes, the same Janice that had tag-teamed with my mom during my horrific formative years. Unfortunately, Janice was just like my mother, but I loved her and wanted a normal sister relationship. I was in awe of her exciting life but understood that inside she was a mess. She had turned to drugs early to numb the pain of our childhood. It was hard to understand how someone who was stunning and brilliant could set out on a journey to destroy herself. Of course, I understood that where we came from was certainly a factor. No one cared about us or showed concern. My mother didn't beat Janice up, but Janice mimicked her behavior. Janice became as mean and hard as my mother.

I used to ask myself, was it because she was first born and was raised by aunts, uncles, grandparents, and parents? She was spoiled rotten it's true. My grandmother used to tell me stories. Regardless of why, she expected her way always. She used her beauty to get what she wanted from everyone, especially men, who acted like lovesick idiots around her. She combined her beauty and brains to convince them to give her money, cars, housing, and jewelry.

I started to really notice something was going on with her when I was around 13 and she was 15. She and I realized that my mother was having an affair with Carl, the man who would become our stepfather. We hated Carl. It wasn't his fault really. We just knew that they were sneaking around and my father didn't know about it. That was a heavy burden for both of us to carry. We discussed telling our father, but he was barely around at this point. We were on our own. I thought Janice was coping. She wasn't.

After our parents divorce, when I was 14 years old, I found Janice in our bathroom with both wrists slit. She was only 16 and already wanted to die. It was her cry for help but no one helped her. What more could I have done as a 14 year old dealing with my own issues? No one spoke of her suicide attempt, ever. All of us should have been in counseling, including my mother, father, and Carl. Instead my parents pretended it never happened. We just carried on. Even I was able to push the incident deep down until all the memories came flooding back as I was writing this book.

I have been in a 12-Step program for years, but this incident didn't surface until I allowed myself to remember at age 69. It is amazing what walls can do to protect our psyche from harm. But so often the pain manifests elsewhere, in my case, in relationships and illness. My sister turned to drugs. I stayed sober so I could get out and save myself. I felt I wasn't smart enough to handle recreational drug use. I needed to stay lucid to survive. I'll talk a lot about my "rules to get through the storms" in the next chapter, but I'll insert one here because it's so important.

**_Gail's Sobriety Rule:_** When things go to hell, stay sober and face life head-on. Don't self-medicate with booze and drugs. There are people and organizations available to help you during tough times and after. I should know, I am in a fabulous 12-Step Program and that is why I am now able to talk about the issues in this book.

Janice left home after high school and went to beauty school. Hairstyling was her love and she was great at it. She was asked to work in Europe with some very famous people. Instead she got a job at the (in)famous Playboy Club in Manhattan. She was "head bunny" at the door. There, she met the men who gave her all she needed. And she also met the man who got her started on hard drugs - Jack Pucino. He was in law school but was a bouncer at the club. He was trouble, and Janice started spiraling downward after she hooked up with him.

Things were ok for a while when Janice and I lived together. We enjoyed a relatively normal sisterly relationship (considering our background and history). We went to all the hot clubs of the era including Studio 54 and

Adam's Apple, and we had good times. We danced all night and I worked all day. I was teaching 3rd, 4th, and 5th grades at a school in Merrick, Long Island and I reverse-commuted for a time while enjoying the New York City nightlife of the 1970s. Life was pretty good. I was still very young. I had a great boyfriend named Tommy with whom I still keep in touch, a good job in a field I absolutely adored, and I got to spend time with my big sister and my little sister. But I hated Janice's boyfriend Jack. The feelings were mutual.

Eventually Janice left the apartment we shared and moved in with Jack. When he got hurt at the club and started taking pain pills, he shared them with Janice. From pain pills like Valium to snorting cocaine, and the rest is history. Janice and Jack got married and started selling drugs together while he was still in law school. That was the eye opener for me. Addicts and dealers come from all walks of life.

I was still dating Tommy and stayed at the apartment Janice and I had rented together in Queens. Tommy and I started what I thought would be a life together, but it didn't work out. I still had paralyzing relationship issues. It would be years before I found stability in that department. Instead of sticking it out with Tommy, in a strange twist of fate, I hooked up with my younger sister Lannie's friend and we took off to Canada! Now I had become the idiot. You can't make this stuff up. Luckily, Lannie has forgiven me for this un-sisterly move and I have forgiven myself for almost ruining my life when it was on the right track.

It turns out the guy was a criminal and I was a kidnapping victim. There's that word again. Victim. What can I say? It's taken many years to break out of that vicious cycle. I was still in my 20s, impressionable, and searching for anyone to show me love, even though at that point I had love. My father came to rescue this time, thankfully, and sent the FBI to retrieve me in Canada and apprehend my criminal companion. Thanks dad! I got away in the nick of time. But while I was making potentially fatal cross-border mistakes, Janice continued to suffer and deteriorate. She stuck with her two favorite things, drugs and Jack.

In 1975 after my kidnapping scare, I moved to South Florida where my father had settled after Puerto Rico, and I was not involved with Janice for a few years. My father was doing well, buying up and developing land in what is today known as Davie, Broward County, Florida. He asked if I would come and work for him. I made that move and I have been in Florida ever since. My life instantly changed with that move. Things were calmer in Florida. I helped my father run his medical building and rode horses in Davie to oversee his orange groves. Working at my dad's company for a year helped me clear my head and reflect on the crazy things I had been doing. My father saved my life by offering me the option of living and working with him, but eventually I had to get out on my own again. I returned to teaching and got my own apartment but stayed in Broward County.

Before I left New York, I knew Janice was still selling drugs and using heavily. I couldn't make her stop. She would have had to leave Jack and get a job. She wasn't ready to do either. It was gut-wrenching to see someone so beautiful and smart self-destruct. But eventually, and miraculously, she did leave Jack and came to me for help in Florida. I sat in a hotel room and watched my sister detox from cocaine, valium, and who knows what else. It took about a week to get her through a full detox, but she made it.

She had enough money from working and dealing in New York, and she decided to stay in Florida and open a clothing store on Biltmore Way in Miami. She opened up "Boobs" and it was a success. For another stretch, life was good. She was a normal sister and we had more fun times. I worked at "Boobs" once a week and loved it. Then one day she announced that she had met a medical student who was working at a local hospital. I didn't think anything of it at the time, certainly not anything bad. But then I met Randy Hrabko.

By this time, in 1979, I was married and was heavily pregnant with my first son Jonathan. He was a spirited mover and kicked me all the time except the day that Randy Hrabko touched my stomach. All the kicking stopped. My unborn child and I were both spooked. Dr. Hrabko was just plain scary. Something about him frightened me and I am not easily scared.

Janice moved in with Dr. Crazy, as I renamed him, and in 1979 he murdered her. I couldn't get anyone to admit that until 2013, when Lannie and I met with Katherine Rundle, State Attorney for Miami-Dade County. We had uncovered enough information to prove he did indeed murder my sister and the police knew it when it happened. He got away with just a drug charge for illegal prescriptions, turned over his Florida medical license, and left the state. He moved to California to practice medicine there. Only if he returned to Florida would he get in trouble.

This was a dark and twisted conspiracy. The police at the time were involved in the selling of drugs that Dr. Randy Hrabko brought in from the Bahamas. They needed him. When I found and interviewed the original medical examiner on Janice's case, he apologized that he had failed her and our family. Janice had two fresh needle marks in her arm, which the medical examiner felt had been skillfully put there by someone in the medical profession. How would Janice have been able to inject herself perfectly with enough morphine to commit suicide, and then be able to make another perfect needle mark with more morphine? She would have been incapacitated at best after the first injection. Not to mention her intense needle phobia, which anyone who knew her well was aware of. So she died, came back to life, and then put another needle in her arm?

Dr. Hrabko had a dead body in his bed yet claimed not to know she was dead. He left the apartment extra early (which he had never done before) saying he thought she was merely sleeping. The woman he supposedly loved, and this complete cluelessness coming from a physician?

I saw the pictures of my dead sister, and the injustice of her murder haunts me to this day. Another wall went up to protect me from that trauma and I didn't talk about it for years. My health took a nosedive after Janice's death and the pain and anger I bottled up inside almost killed me. Years later Dr. Harbko lost his own daughter to a drug overdose. Now he knows the agony of losing someone so dear. Welcome to my world Dr. Harbko.

Prior to Janice's murder I had a few healthy years. I swam, ran, and played tennis. My Florida lifestyle was healthy and I felt ok. I was still young, so able to stave off disease. Lannie also came down to Florida to live with me, which was great. I had married the father of my two sons in 1978. Ronnie Dvoretz was a man I had met in the apartment complex where I lived. I got pregnant immediately after we married. But this was not a good match. I was still in an unhealthy relationship pattern. I married and replaced my mother, except he was the male version.

Before Jonathon was born, my mother also decided to move down to Florida in an attempt to have a relationship with her first grandchild, and I assume, me. Talk about the perfect storm: a bad marriage, the murder of my sister, and the return of the woman who had tormented me from birth. Dysfunction and tragedy transplanted from New York to Florida. This was the beginning of the end of my physical health as well as my mental health.

What should have been a wonderful time in a new mother's life became a horror to me. My husband Ronnie was a cold and callous human being. After my sister was killed, he generously offered his opinion on the matter. "You are better off without Janice. She was a scumbag!" You can imagine how that affected our relationship. Janice was imperfect, no one knew that more than me, but she was my sister and I loved her. I never forgave his remark and the relationship steadily deteriorated.

My first autoimmune disease struck in 1979 right after Jonathan was born. I was gaining weight and could hardly hold up my new baby. I had no concern or support from Ronnie. I was alone and sick. It was Hashimoto's disease and I was eventually put on thyroid pills and they helped me lose the weight and gain back some energy. However, by then my feelings for Ronnie had changed. My marriage was on the rocks and I was stressed and depressed.

My second son Brett was born in 1981 and that same year I was diagnosed as a diabetic (originally misdiagnosed as a type 2 and later correctly as a brittle type 1). I almost died from blood sugars topping 900 and a very bad flu. I was determined not to go down without a fight, but by then, the marriage was unbearable (it finally ended in 1984), and I was caring for two small sons with a husband who wasn't really interested in anyone but himself. So now I had my bipolar mother around to remind me of my miserable past, a murdered sister for whom I couldn't get justice, and a narcissistic ex-husband to torment me. The mental health problems had gotten their foot in my door and it wasn't long before the physical health followed. I now had two serious autoimmune diseases. They were getting ready to knock the house down. If you had given me a preview of what I would be facing over the next few decades, I might have asked you to let me bail right then and there, but I tend to get on with things and fight back. Thanks mom!

# 4

# GAIL'S RULES FOR GETTING THROUGH THE STORMS

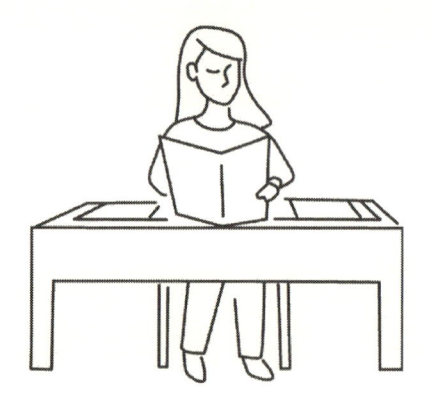

In 1983, at the age of 34, I was arrested for driving under the influence of drugs or alcohol. I was under the influence of neither. I was only guilty of driving under the assumption that my doctor knew how to treat diabetes…and assuming that all cops were good and only arrested bad people. I was wrong on both counts. My endocrinologist at the time had failed to explain what low blood sugar was and that severely low blood sugar could occur when taking the new drug he had prescribed. He had also failed to explain what low blood sugar felt like or looked like. Apparently, it looked like a DUI.

The officer who arrested me failed to see that I was a very scared and sick woman. She failed to protect me and instead chose to beat me up, throw me in jail, plant drugs on me, and refuse to acknowledge that I was ill and in need of help.

That terrible experience prompted me to develop what I call **Gail's Rules** (remember Gail's Sobriety Rule? There's more!).

***Gail's Rule Number One***: Don't blindly trust police officers. At the end of the day they are human. They jump to conclusions and make mistakes. They can beat you up and lock you away if they want to, even if you are completely innocent. They did it to me, so I know. Jail is not fun for sick people. My dad saved my life again. He came to the jail and told the cops what was happening.

***Gail's Rule Number Two***: Don't think that doctors know everything because if you do you are in big trouble. Doctors are also human. They read medical books and then practice what they read or learned from other doctors that wrote and read the very same books. They make mistakes and they are stubborn.

I have only two doctors that I trust and adore. One, Dr. Ross, I call "God." He's an old-fashioned doctor who actually thinks before he writes prescriptions. He is a generational physician. He took care of my mother, me, my sister, and my children. The few doctors left like him are the last of the great diagnosticians. Without Dr. Ross I would have been sick for a long time. The other one is also very special to me. I found Dr. Kenny Tourgemen, a kidney specialist, because of my diabetes. I didn't know he was really a holistic physician. Years later when everyone was calling me crazy, (one of the many times I've been called crazy!), and I walked into Dr. Kenny's office, something wonderful happened. He listened. He took one look at me and told me to stop eating bagels. I told him I hadn't had a bagel in three months. I told him I was gluten free. He said I was doing the right thing. I looked up in tears and knew I had found the doctor I needed. That was a decade ago, long before going gluten free became fashionable. I am pretty sure that I had acquired as much information about my diseases as my endocrinologist and now needed help from a doctor who knew about this mystery substance that was killing both Lannie and me.

Little did I know how many people suffer from gluten intolerance and still go undiagnosed because doctors are not trained in nutrition. But I learned by reading as many books as possible about all of my medical conditions. I say "my" because I own them. I was willing to give up those bagels and donuts and do anything to control my diabetes. I was (and am) also willing to do anything to prevent the loss of my eyesight, legs, or kidneys from diabetic complications. In order to survive I became a diabetic specialist and continue to follow an aggressive plan for treating it.

Many of my doctors thought that my methods were *too* aggressive. I was ridiculed when I started taking insulin shots as needed to control it. I was years ahead of the medical community. I was performing what they now call "Aggressive Insulin Therapy" 20 years before the medical community even thought of it. Yes, it now has a name. And the very same doctors who told me that what I was doing was not necessary were wrong, and they are now promoting this very therapy. But how many lives have they affected negatively by putting their heads in the sand?

*__Gail's Rule Number Three__:* Any person with any disease should be wearing a Medic Alert bracelet or necklace and be signed up with that company (www.MedicAlert.org). There are a number of excellent companies that provide necklaces and bracelets. They are inexpensive and can save your life. I have a few necklaces in silver and black and I purchase at least five of them for the year. To be honest, I lose them all the time. I leave them everywhere, so I need back-ups. Regardless, I need them, and if you have any diseases, you need them.

*__Gail's Rule Number Four__:* Get some strategies to deal with stress. Meditation is one good way and joining some kind of support group to help you cope is another. The human body can only handle so much stress before it begins to break down like mine did. Learning how to handle stress should be a required high school class. Life is full of stressors and triggers, and if we mishandle them, we risk ending up irreparably damaged.

Within a week of my arrest, my blood sugar shot straight up and never came down again. My body was in a constant state of fear. I was afraid to drive because of my low blood sugar experience (ironically because now it was always sky high) and I panicked every time I saw a police officer. All this stress was pushing my immune system into hell and this is when it went into overdrive. My then-husband Ronnie and I were not doing well, which added to the trauma. Things like illnesses and death can push an already troubled marriage past the point of no return. By 1984 we were divorced and it was the right thing to do. If I had stayed with him I would be dead by now. So looking back, divorcing Ron was a gift because shortly after my divorce I met and married Larry. We've been together for over 30 years.

## Type 1 Diabetes

I went to the doctor after my run-in with the law, and he admitted that he had made a mistake. I was not a type 2 diabetic, but instead a type 1. If you know anything about diabetes, you know that type 1 is MUCH more complicated than type 2. I <u>didn't</u> know. Years later I realized that if that doctor had put me on insulin right away I might have salvaged some of my islet cells. Islets (pronounced EYE-lets) are clusters of cells in the pancreas that work together to regulate blood sugars. Within these cell clusters are cells that detect sugar in the blood and release insulin to maintain normal blood sugar levels. The immune system of a type 1 diabetic sees these cells as dangerous and destroys them. Healthy islets can be transplanted into a diabetic pancreas and have been found to work normally for twelve years. I could have used my functioning islet cells now when I need them.

When it was confirmed by the almighty medical establishment that I was a type 1 insulin dependent brittle diabetic, I went to Holy Cross Hospital in Fort Lauderdale and enrolled in a stupid and uninformative class about how to take shots and treat my new disease. They suggested only two shots a day. I thought that was a joke. At my first class, I told the nurse *not* to give me a shot in the stomach because I would pass out. She didn't believe me, which is too bad because as soon as she injected me in the stomach, I gracefully passed out. A severe fear of needles began with that first shot. I was never able to take shots in my stomach because I could see the needles going in. It was bad enough taking shots anywhere in my body. Like all, and I mean ALL type 1 diabetics, I was put on a two shot per day regime. This did nothing to control the disease and my frustration with the medical community continued.

Dr. Biederman, my endocrinologist, was constantly yelling at me for both my weight gain and my seeming inability to control this disease. No matter how hard I tried on their program, I failed. I would use the urine strips and hope for the color blue. If the strip was not blue, I would go out and run. If I couldn't run, I would bounce on a small trampoline at night in my house. Sometimes at one or two in the morning when I saw the brown strip, I would start to exercise and still go teach the next day. It was horrible. If I hadn't changed my protocol, this story would not have been written.

A "type 1 brittle diabetic," is also known as an "out of control type 1." I realized what that meant. It meant that no one understood my disease. It meant that no matter what I did, I was going to struggle to control it. Regardless, I was still willing to go at it every single day. I rarely ate "junk" food. I exercised all day long, any time of the day or night, to keep my blood sugar levels below 110. These numbers were unheard of in the diabetic community but for me that number was my goal. I taught myself discipline with food. Do I cheat once in a while? Yes. I am human. But I do so infrequently, and I always cover anything high in sugar or carbs with insulin or exercise or both.

Life went on in the 80s and for some years nothing too stressful entered into my life except for dealing with brittle type 1 diabetes every single day, mourning my sister's murder, holding down a job, and caring for two small sons. Add all that to the nightmare that had been my early life, and the recipe for bad health had put a stamp on me. My gut was injured and that is where all the bad (and good) stuff originates. Who knew? Wait, I thought doctors knew. Again, I was so wrong, and it was only a matter of time until more stress came my way and I was not ready for it. It was my health again, and things were really going to heat up.

By the time I was 40 (1989) I had three autoimmune diseases, diabetes type 1, vitiligo, where you lose skin pigment, and Hashimotos thyroid disease, where the thyroid is under-active. I had been taking Synthroid to replace what my thyroid used to do for me, and insulin to replace my pancreas, but I lost all my pigment and turned white. Most of my life I had been olive skinned and tan, but now I looked like Snow White. There is no replacement for lost pigment, only a few treatments, but because my body was in overdrive, treatment didn't work.

I was hoping that this unholy autoimmune disease trinity would be it. I had what is now called poly-glandular failure and that seemed like plenty. I like to call it "one-too-many-autoimmune-diseases." I had asked my doctor how many diseases I could get and he knowingly lied to me and said only three. I loved him for lying to me but I learned the hard way that I could get many more. My sister Lannie was not doing well either. We both were hit hard by the autoimmune dysfunction but I wasn't sure why it was happening to both of us.

My father contributed a few of his own rules right before he died of bone marrow cancer in 1990. He said, "Gail if you want to make it in this world you had better become your own doctor and your own lawyer." I laughed at him then but now I know he was right. Eventually I took those words to heart without even realizing it. Sadly he didn't fare as well as I did. He didn't take his own advice and he died from inflammation of his heart, bone cancer, and not controlling his diabetes. His cancer was in remission but his heart couldn't handle the stress of the drugs. His death and the way he died was another hit to the Keehn sisters' immune systems.

Right after my father passed away Lannie came down with chronic fatigue syndrome and fibromyalgia, both autoimmune diseases, and both completely debilitating. Lannie too had poly-glandular failure. She had Hashimotos, adrenal gland failure, chronic fatigue/ fibromyalgia, a weird autoimmune disease that wiped out her ovaries, IBS (irritable bowel syndrome), heartburn, and more. We were both suffering, and I mean really suffering.

Autoimmune diseases can drag you down to zero quality of life. I had to get smart and figure out what was ***really*** going on. Like a research scientist/detective, I vowed to get to the bottom of what was happening. It would take more stress and even more autoimmune diseases for me to finally figure it out.

# 5

# DIABETES – ACCEPT AND CONQUER

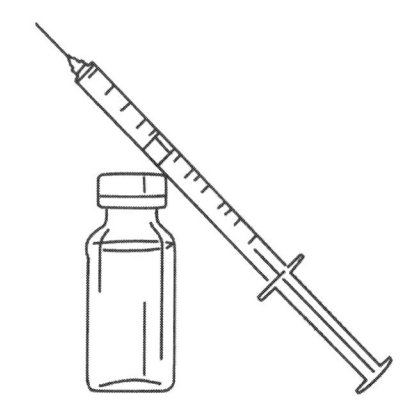

So, I made it to age 37 trying to follow the American diabetes diet and without medical help or any direction from the medical community, it was becoming more and more difficult to control the disease. I had no understanding of how the human body worked. I had dropped out of biology at Nassau Community College, and because of my lack of biology knowledge, I was at a major disadvantage when it came to helping myself.

***Gail's Rule Number Five***: Stay in school and take all those classes; even the ones you hate and think you won't use. You never know when you might actually need all that weird and "useless" information. I needed to understand the function of a pancreas in order to live and keep all my body parts but didn't know it when I bailed out of biology.

Instead of letting myself remain at the mercy of the medical establishment, I went back to college for biology. I didn't take the class for credit and didn't cut up any baby pigs for a grade, which was the reason I had dropped the class in the first place. I just went for the knowledge of how the pancreas worked within the human body. I also wanted to understand autoimmune diseases and what was causing my body to fail. During that class I learned enough to figure out what I had to do to control this monster of a disease. I had to emulate the pancreas with my needle in hand and so I did. Again, against medical advice I started to take way more shots but took less and less insulin. I now had no unused insulin floating inside my body. I only took what I needed and didn't have to eat to keep up with the stupid "two large doses in shots a day" regimen. However, year after year of taking five to ten shots a day I was becoming needle phobic again. Can you imagine how awful it was? Someone who absolutely hates needles. I really struggled to take those shots but I kept at it so I could keep my blood sugars normal. I had children and wanted to be there for them. Doctors were always amazed at my diabetic control, but when I shared how I was doing it, they ignored me or told me I was crazy. I was right then, and I am still on earth to prove it. No diabetic complications and I keep on dancing.

I was always looking for ways to improve my insulin regimen. One day my mom, (remember she moved to Florida before Jonathan was born in 1979), happily called and said she had seen something on TV that talked about a needle-free syringe. She actually helped me that day, but I figure she owed me! She hadn't taken the name of the company or the phone number, but she was excited to tell me nonetheless. I began my research to find it at any cost. After many phone calls (this was pre-Google) I discovered the company was called MEDI-JECTOR. I went back to Dr. Biederman and naively asked for a prescription to get this wonderful life saving technology. What was his response? He told me it didn't work. I asked him how he knew that. We stared at each other and I finally stood up and said, "You, doctor, are an idiot. You have a client in front of you who is taking needles all day long and keeping her diabetes under control. You don't know a thing about this technology, and you are lying to me." I handed him the 70 needles that I had brought to his office. They were in my bag and I told him to stick himself like I did for just one week to see how he liked it. After that we could talk intelligently. I was no longer going to listen to a doctor who was dismissing and condescending to all people with diabetes. His protocol was the same for every patient, regardless of their individual differences, and he expected a different result. That, we know, is insanity. I was neither insane nor stupid. The medical community was living in the dark ages with regard to treating diabetes and I was no longer going to be part of that life. I was not going to be one more of its victims. I walked out of Dr. Biederman's office and never looked back.

Three weeks later I actually found a good doctor in Fort Lauderdale who agreed that we had nothing to lose by trying this new needle-less technology. He acknowledged that all of the shots I was taking were keeping my strips a beautiful blue so what did I have to lose by doing the same thing but without needles? He wrote the prescription I so badly needed. I had to spend $1,200 on my very first Medi-Jector, and it was worth every penny. I began using the first needle-free insulin delivery system ever seen in the world. I was one of their first clients. I have not looked back since and because of this treatment I have no complications from a disease that kills or maims almost everyone who gets it. That is not to say that my diabetes isn't a constant battle. It is. But I don't give up.

***Addendum to Gail's Rule Number Two***: Doctors are <u>not</u> Gods. They are human beings. They can be close-minded to new treatments and see themselves as superior to their patients. They are mistaken. Even though they take an oath to "do no harm," they are often unable to see the forest for the trees. The end result is needless suffering and even premature death. Be your own health advocate. Don't listen to them if it doesn't feel right. Fight for yourself and for those you love.

After years of floundering alone with a terrible and treacherous disease, I learned that I needed to take ownership of the cards I was dealt. I made it my job to read and study and learn and stay informed on things coming down the pike that might help my unique situation. I learned to treat myself and to choose health. My doctors might not care about my limbs, but I was determined to keep all of my body parts intact.

.

6

# THE MEDI-JECTOR – CHANGING THE COURSE OF MY DISEASE

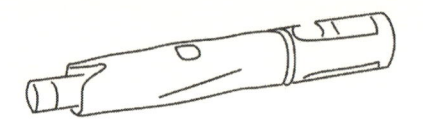

I was ecstatic when I received the prescription I needed to order the Medi-Jector. It seemed odd to me that no one else had heard about the FDA passing such a wonderful device. Now, years later, I fully understand the process. Sadly, I have learned what the FDA did (and still do) and with whom they are in cahoots. It wasn't and isn't the people they are supposed to represent. They are in business with Big Pharma, not the average U.S. citizen. They do not look out for the safety or well-being of the people of this country. I could say it is just because they are stupid and ignorant, but I think the truth is more sinister.

**Gail's Rule Number Six:** Don't believe the FDA because the FDA is FOS (Full of S*#t). *See Chapter 8.*

Before I got my Medi-Jector, I decided I would reserve judgment before reviewing it and recommending it to other diabetics. It was delivered while my mother and Lannie were at my house in Coral Springs, Florida. Meanwhile I was jabbing myself somewhere between 8-15 times a day with needles. I had black and blue arms from all of my shots. It was just a never-ending nightmare. We know how I feel about shots in the stomach, they're not happening. What I had left were my arms, legs, and butt. All bad choices, but I had to do it. The day the mailman delivered the box, I just sat there looking at it and praying that this was the real deal. Before I even opened it, I ran upstairs, took all my needles except three, and walked out the door to my garbage bins. My mother grabbed my arm and said, "Gail, what are you doing with those needles? Give them to me." I looked up crying and said, "I am sorry mom, but if this doesn't work, I don't want to be here anymore." It sounds dramatic but I meant it. I knew what the future held if I didn't find something different. I saw people at the hospital with no legs. I saw people waiting for dialysis, many of them blind. I couldn't put my family through that suffering. I didn't want to put myself through it. I wanted to be remembered as strong and vibrant. If the Medi-Jector didn't work, I was planning my exit.

Looking back, I realize how very selfish I was. My mother had already lost one daughter and her other two were suffering with illness. I shouldn't have shown my despair. To her credit, my mother let go of my hand and sat down on the garage floor and let me just cry.

I went back into the house, opened my new needle-less insulin delivery system, and read the directions. I was scared to death and decided to watch the video that came with it. I think I watched it at least eight times before I went to the kitchen to sterilize the parts that needed to be cleaned. I took one more needle that night because I had to wait for the system to dry. The next morning I took my first shot without a needle and never looked back. In my hand I had another prescription for another machine so if it worked I wouldn't have to wait for my machine to dry, or in case the first one broke.

My miracle happened. I knew I had done the right thing. Years later when the pump came out, it became the "big thing" in treating type 1 diabetes. It allowed patients to take multiple injections as needed. The medical community had finally caught up with me but it took them 15 long years. Doctors were finally telling patients to do what I had already been doing and promoting. I had saved my own life and all my body parts. My Medi-Jector was my pancreas. Thirty plus years later I am still using it, but nobody else can get it because they stopped producing it.

Amazingly, in 2014 the company took it off the market due to lack of sales. I had purchased enough supplies to last me the rest of my life, but nobody else could. There were not enough kickbacks or money in that treatment. They never told people about the needle-less insulin delivery system for decades, because they never bothered to understand how it worked. This is not unusual in our country, but it is tragic and criminal. Some Medi-Jector alternatives have come on the market, and since 2017, needle free insulin delivery systems are booming, finally. But all those years and all those patients who never knew about the Medi-Jector and continued to suffer with needles. I can't even think about it without getting infuriated all over again.

**_Gail's Rule Number Seven:_** Don't trust that big business is working for you. They are not. We are all just dollar signs. We must take control of our lives and our health. I can't repeat that enough times.

7

# IT AIN'T EASY, BUT MAKE FOOD YOUR FRIEND

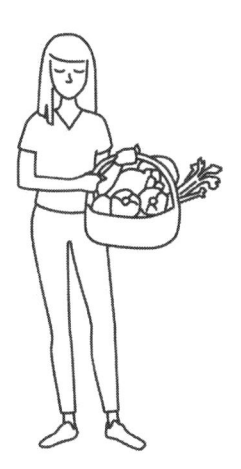

My amazing Medi-Jector essentially served as my new pancreas, so I could manage my blood sugar highs in a single shot whenever I needed to without the needles. The next part of the learning curve was just as important and required even more research and discipline. Something so many of us have trouble managing, understanding, and controlling, and something that we all need help with: food.

Prior to finger-pricking technology, I had urinated on strips to keep track of my blood sugar. This was not effective in really taking charge of my disease because the readings would only show what my blood sugar was two hours before. I had never been a fan of the strips and knew that something better had to come along. Frankly, I thought they were ridiculous, but the medical establishment encouraged me to use them. Finally, finger-pricking put my readings in "real time" and although it's no fun to prick your finger a dozen times a day, losing limbs, eyes, or kidneys is less fun. With this technology, I could analyze how everything I put in my mouth affected my blood sugar. Again, I took on the role of guinea pig. With a notebook in one hand and a glucose meter in the other, I was ready to dig in and figure this one out. What foods affected my blood sugar? How long did it stay high before it came down below 110.

My husband suggested that I record every meal I had. I would eat, test, and write the results in my notebook. I would test at the 30-minute mark, then one hour, and then two. In about a week we figured out that potatoes, pizza, rice, and any other complex carb would shoot my blood sugars way up. Even bananas had the same effect, as did too much protein. I found these experiments fascinating. Through trial and error, I was learning how and what to eat to keep my blood sugars tightly controlled. As usual, this was all up to me, and not my doctors. By this time, I had learned that I was the only who could take the credit if my plan worked, or the blame if it didn't. Meaningful guidance from anyone in the medical community would have been nice, but it was not to be found.

After one month of testing and writing it down my husband and I came up with an eating plan. I wouldn't eat carbs unless I was going to exercise or it was daytime and I could work it off. Back then I was mostly vegetarian, so many of those carb choices had to be addressed. I only ate fish, cheese, and eggs for protein, so restricting carbs was tough. I was willing to do it. I sat down with my notebook and planned out my new lifestyle diet. It was then that everything changed.

***Gail's Rule Number Eight***: Learn to live with hunger or drink lots of hot tea and broths that contain things like spinach, kale, onions, and cabbage. Those foods don't raise blood sugar. Save high carbs like beans, rice, and potatoes for the morning run or bike ride and don't eat them after 4:00 p.m., unless you are going to exercise in the evening. Those carbs must be used as a fuel.

My life began to feel more manageable as I took control of my eating and really took the time to write everything down. I lost the weight I had gained while on the diabetic diet recommended by the medical establishment. Breakfast was a vegetable omelet with a side of salad or chicken with vegetables. Lunch was my carb time and it usually included one serving of potato, rice, or beans and a protein like tofu or fish and a vegetable or salad. Dinner was the same as lunch without the complex carbs. I always had three snacks a day. They usually consisted of a piece of fruit or cookies that I made with some type of weird flour. (Check out the *Recipes* section of this book or my website, www.GlutenFreeGail.com, for lots of meal ideas). I ate ice cream but only in small servings. Every Sunday I gave myself a break and threw caution to the wind. I ate what I wanted but always pricked my finger to see if I needed more insulin or if my blood sugar was out of control.

I now had a diet plan to go with my diabetes treatment. Today, 35 years later, my idea of a great dinner is eggplant baked in slices with a smattering of tuna fish on top. I snack throughout the day on sliced peppers, celery, cucumbers, chopped up lettuce in chunks and small cherry tomatoes. I love vegetables and make them the centerpiece of my nutrition. Instead of feeling deprived and miserable because I can't pig out, I feel great. I didn't die from making those food sacrifices all those years ago. I began to live. They don't feel at all like sacrifices anymore. Sometimes on my "fun" days my blood sugar spikes, but I don't get too worried about it since high blood sugar once in awhile won't do that much harm. I just make sure it doesn't stay high for too long.

For a while I was quite the happy camper on this diet. I thought I was in complete control of my life. I had given up what I thought I needed to and managed to prevent the complications I saw other diabetics around me dealing with. Unfortunately, I saw some diabetic friends become quite ill and even die from these complications, including my father. At the time my only question was, would I stay healthy? Only time would tell.

## Mary Kay

As I think back on my life between 1983 and 2009 – when the bulk of my health problems manifested, I am amazed to remember the many things I managed to do successfully, despite so many setbacks. My experience with Mary Kay is one of those. I went outside of my comfort zone and dared to try something that scared me to death, and it paid off.

In the early 90s, I was always struggling to make ends meet as a teacher. I worked all year round and tutored on Saturdays. There was never enough money to survive on a teaching salary. Larry and I both found extra jobs to help support my two kids and his two kids. Special-Ed tutors do not make a lot of money on the side – but what else was I going to do?

In 1994 I was asked to go to a Mary Kay party. I had never heard of Mary Kay, but my friends had. They tried to dissuade me from attending. They were worried that I would be forced to sign up. As soon as they expressed those fears, I don't know why, but I decided to attend anyway and dragged Lannie with me. I wanted to see what they were talking about - what could be so bad about makeup, perfume, and body soaps? Plus I was always ready for a party.

When we got there we saw beautiful women in red jackets sitting at the front of the room. A Sales Director named Pam led the meeting. She was my eventual recruiter (and still very high in the company even today). While there I thought, make-up and money? I can do this. So after getting make-up put on my face and having a wonderful evening I signed up and so did Lannie. I guess my friends were right. But it wasn't by force. I was intrigued by the thought of supplementing my income helping women take care of their skin and look pretty.

As usual, my supportive husband smiled when I told him what I had just done. Lannie's husband however made fun of her and hurt her feelings. Like I said, she married our mother!

Because my kids were young teenagers and no longer interested in playing or spending time with me, I decided to turn any free time I had into money. I set up my kitchen so that people could sit at a table and try on makeup and skin care items. I had so much fun. I began to sell a lot of product and before I knew it I was recruiting other women and training them to do what I was doing. I made sure all of my classes were held in my home so I could watch my kids. Within one month of selling, I told Larry that I wanted to become a Mary Kay Director. He encouraged me to do whatever makes me happy and go for it. Three months later I had become a Mary Kay Director with a 50-person unit and won my first Pontiac Firebird.

I believed everything Mary Kay promoted: God first, Family second, Business third. I had a family and a full-time teaching job, so I didn't have a lot of extra time on my hands, but I made it work. However, this is where I made a mistake. Lannie was shy and was not interested in recruiting people. I did her recruiting for her and added another 50 women to her unit and won a car for her too. So, I ended up doing all the work for both of us and that is almost impossible to sustain. Had I not started the unit for my sister I am convinced I'd be a National Sales Director today. This is one of the reasons I needed to be in a 12-step program. It's ok to help people, as long as it doesn't hurt you. But who knows if I would have stuck with it even though I was a natural at sales and recruiting.

At the huge company convention in Dallas, I learned that Mary Kay was a multilevel marketing company with a few big wigs at the top of the pyramid making all the money and the little people at the bottom doing all of the hard work and hardly making anything. I did all the training and recruiting for the whole unit and had to maintain sales quotas in order to keep the car. As unit members quit, I'd have to replace them or lose my status. It was constant pressure. I was a bit disillusioned to find out about the structure of the company, but I can honestly say that I did have a blast going to Dallas, getting up on stage to get my award and recognition, and meeting Mary Kay.

When I won my car I had to speak on stage in Dallas, so I quickly got over my fear of speaking to a massive audience. I am forever grateful to Mary Kay for giving me a vehicle (no pun intended) to discover my speaking potential and my selling potential! I didn't get a pink Cadillac, however, because that required way more team members and way more product sold. If I had just focused on my own team building, I would have gotten that Cadillac. But in those days I didn't just look after myself, I always looked after Lannie too. And I'm glad I did it that way. Our road trip to Dallas via New

Orleans and our time at the national Mary Kay headquarters is a memory I cherish. But self-care is a top priority for me now and it should be for you too.

***Gail's Self-Care Rule***: Take care of yourself and the rest will follow. Put your oxygen mask on first, then you can help others. If you don't put yourself first, your health, both mental and physical, will suffer. Despite my success, I was not healthy in my head or my body. I was still trying to fix me. I just hadn't learned how to do it properly.

My Mary Kay career actually ended tragically. We suffered a house fire, and my entire inventory (thousands of dollars worth) literally went up in smoke. The woman who recruited me didn't advise me to purchase inventory insurance in the event of fire, flood, theft, etc. I lost everything. That's also when I discovered the not-so-Godly side of Mary Kay. They were not very kind when I needed to replace my inventory. They just wanted me to spend thousands to repurchase everything. There was no way I was going to do that. Since I wasn't selling and recruiting, I wasn't important anymore.

I would never encourage women to join a multilevel marketing company unless they are gifted in sales, are not shy to recruit other team members, and are willing to put in some serious hours. But I did learn a lot on my Mary Kay journey. Until then, I had never felt I was good at anything, even with my hard-earned degrees and my teaching job. I still bore the scars of my mother's abuse. It is no secret that children are more likely to be successful and well-adjusted if they grow up with accepting and loving parents. Wealth is less important than love and kindness. I never had those things, so I was never kind to myself. Despite everything, I still saw a fat girl, an ugly woman, and someone without any brains. But with each new endeavor - and I include Mary Kay - I gained confidence.

Lannie once said to me, "I would rather mom hit me than continue the verbal torture." It's a sad choice, but I agree with her. The mind-body-health connection is real. A sick mind makes an unhealthy body. My sister and I are proof of that. I had to work through so much, but now, at age 70, I know who Gail is and I'm proud of her. The girl who never thought she was good at anything obviously was. I just had to see and acknowledge her.

Mary Kay also taught me how speak publicly with authority, which in turn helped me speak at an FDA meeting and at the White House in 1996. Had I not signed that Mary Kay agreement, I would never have had the courage to speak in front of 500 people in chairs behind me and a panel of eminent endocrinologists in front of me. I would never have gone to the White House to speak on behalf of all of our nation's diabetics. More on that next chapter.

***Gail's Self-Love Rule***: Learn to love yourself and be accepting of yourself as you are. You are the most important person in your life. And if you have to do a presentation in front of hundreds of people, picturing them naked really works!

# 8

# THE FDA IS FOS

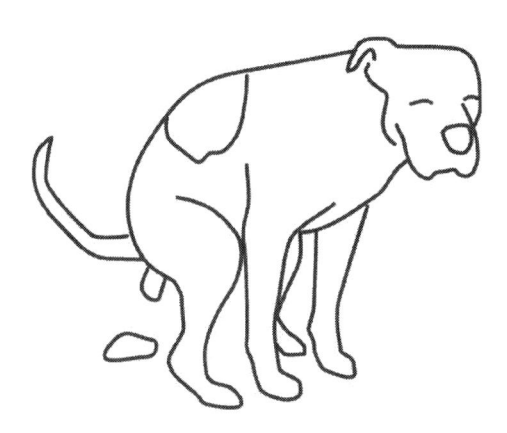

My father once said that if I lived long enough, eventually they would find cures for whatever diseases I had.

**_Gail's Rule Number Nine:_** Don't wait for any disease to be cured. There is way too much money in treatment. The days of the polio vaccine are gone and so are the ethics behind finding a cure. Now there is Big Pharma. They don't want to cure diabetes, cancer, or **anything** that would interfere with their money-making obsession.

In 1996 I had the opportunity to see this for myself. I was invited to speak at an FDA convention to help bring a new technology to the diabetic community. I was always searching for information about the latest advancements in diabetes management and I found out a company called Biocontrol Technology was going to an FDA oversight hearing to get approval for their new device, the Diasensor. At the time, I naively believed that if something was wonderful for a sick population, it was the FDA's job to make sure it reached those people. I was wrong.

The Diasensor was supposed to be the first non-invasive glucose meter. That meant no more strips and no more finger pricks to determine blood glucose levels. I had been watching Biocontrol and their technology for about two years and was waiting for the product to come out so I could use it. I was unaware of the FDA's process to grant approval for a new technology. I called Biocontrol Technology and asked when they were going to go to the FDA hearing. Diane McQuaid, the company PR representative, informed me that they were preparing for the hearing. I offered my assistance as a person who was pricking their finger 16 times per day, and had for years. I asked if I could get up and speak about how this new technology would save many lives and would change my life forever. Ms. McQuaid accepted my offer to speak so I called the FDA and told them I wanted to do a presentation. I must have sounded a bit flaky. I was so busy with my life, I'm not sure I made much sense. The FDA contact agreed to put me down as one of the speakers, probably thinking I wouldn't make a positive impression and didn't know what I was talking about.

Their attitude changed a week before the meeting when I called back to get the schedule and confirm my time slot. All of a sudden, the same FDA contact started trying to dissuade me from coming to Maryland. She must have realized that I was not the idiot I had sounded like in the prior conversation, and that I was serious and had my act together. She asked why I wanted this technology and tried to convince me that I really didn't need it because I had my condition under control. I wondered briefly why she would do that, but eventually I called back and confirmed I was coming and to put me down for 30 minutes. You could have heard a pin drop on the other end of the line.

I put the awkward conversation aside and was excited to find out how the FDA worked. Once Larry and I arrived at the hotel, I put the final touches on my presentation. I was still teaching at the time and I decided to approach this opportunity as though I were presenting at a science fair, just like my students. I wanted to emphasize old technology vs. new technology and the benefits of every new development to the life of a type 1 diabetic. I went "full-on educator mode" and used panel displays and magic markers in my presentation. I explained about the "way things used to be," "where we are now," and "where we need to go."

I got my chance to speak and presented to an audience of more than 500 people, many of them sick diabetics, as well as 20 of the leading endocrinologists in the U.S. During my presentation, the doctors were very arrogant. They had the nerve to suggest that pricking your finger "doesn't really hurt." Of course it doesn't hurt…them! But if you prick your finger several times daily, believe me, it hurts. But me telling them wasn't enough. I needed to show them that daily finger pricking DID hurt.

"So gentleman," I said. "I have explained why the technology needs to go forward. Complacency has set in. If you don't think that pricking fingers everyday hurts, we are now going to hand out the lancets I use all day long. I want you to all prick your fingers. Not just once. I want you to stick yourself 15 times and let's see how you like it." I then asked, "how many of you are diabetic and can relate to what I am saying?" A quiet hush engulfed the panel. Not one of the panel doctors had diabetes. I waited as they tried over and over to prick their fingers. Only one could actually do it, but the machine read "Not Enough Blood." I told him he would need to prick his finger again in order to get more blood. He said he couldn't do it. "Well," I said, "we as diabetics don't have the option of *not* doing it. If we choose not to finger prick, we risk dying." I emphasized loudly that that was why this technology *needed* to pass to help it go forward and positively impact the daily life of diabetics. I was very naïve. I was about to learn how the government and the Food & Drug Administration ran our country.

The panel decided **not** to approve the Diasensor even though it was available in the European Union and was being used all day long by diabetics who loved it and were eternally grateful not to have to prick their fingers. The only thing the diabetic community in the U.S. needed was for that first machine to be passed. The funding to bring the next generation of the Diasensor was already set to go forward. It just needed the first approval. But the FDA turned it down. They simply didn't care. They didn't prick their fingers – their diabetic patients did, and who cared about them? I was in shock. I came to find out that nine out of the 20 panel doctors owned stock in the companies that made the finger pricking strips.

I was devastated by this failure. I had done given it my all. I had explained to the panel of experts how many times I pricked my fingers in one day, which was 12-16 times and how that translated to about 5,475 times per year. I had asked them to do the same just once. I had handed out statistics on diabetes for everyone. There were people in that audience, diabetics, who had lost eyesight and limbs. There were people holding tubes because their kidneys were failing. I knew from my research that sometimes diabetics lose control of their disease because constant finger pricking hurts so much, they chose not to do it. Or worse, they were willing to withstand the pain, but their insurance companies would only pay for 200 strips per month and they required many more. These people needed this technology to be approved. They needed it desperately, but that didn't matter. What mattered to those panel doctors was the big money their companies made on testing strips and they were not going to put them out of business.

Unfortunately, Biocontrol Technology could never deliver on the Diasensor and I am still pricking my fingers to this day. After the FDA hearing, the head of the company, Fred Cooper, faced merciless scrutiny and was made out to be the bad guy. He was accused of falsifying reports and duping shareholders. It is my firm belief that he was set up. The FDA would not approve the device and he was destroyed as a result.

On the ride home from Maryland, I wept because I had learned the hard way that there would not be a cure or a treatment that would genuinely help people with diabetes unless it made money for the investors and Big Pharma. I haven't seen anything new or different for the treatment of type 1 diabetes from the time I was diagnosed in 1981 until now, 38 years later. Yes, they do have the pump but that is still a needle. You need to be on the pump to have a needle-less blood-testing device attached. I wanted no needles. They do have the OmniPod but again, that is something sticking into me.

After my presentation, some people did come over to talk to me about my needle-less insulin delivery system, my wonderful Medi-Jector. Their doctors had never told them about it. Only one endocrinologist came over to see how I was taking needle-less shots. The rest of them didn't care about that either, even though I had showed them the technology during my presentation. Many hadn't heard of it and didn't want to know.

From that point on I knew that if I wanted to live with this disease, I was on my own. I knew this already, but it was constantly being reinforced. Their attitude was "who gives a crap?" These were the best doctors in the US. Can you imagine what the worst ones were like?

For me it was even more difficult to find a knowledgeable doctor because when the patient knows more than the doctor, who needs a doctor? Unfortunately, I need doctors for prescriptions to get insulin. But I didn't ask an endocrinologist to help me treat my disease until 2016 when I met the second endocrinologist I could trust enough to look at my testing device and give me suggestions on how to prevent my blood sugar lows. At first, I told her she was not going to treat my diabetes. She could only treat my thyroid. As time went on I began to trust Dr. Krysiak. She understood the importance of staying gluten free when you have type 1 or type 2 diabetes. That was enough for me. She got it!

We talked about the new thyroid medication I wanted to try. She actually had it in her office and gave me a free two-month supply. I had found my doctor. For the first time in my diabetic life I handed over my testing machine so a doctor could look at it and give me advice. I cried in her office and she understood. It is a hard disease to do alone and I had done it alone for decades. She actually knew more than I did. I made jokes about that because I had never met a doctor who knew more than I did.

**<u>Addendum to Gail's Rule Number Six</u>**: Don't trust the FDA. They are not in business for the people they serve. They are in business for Big Pharma and are controlled by Big Pharma and other big corporations that are not in business to help people either.

9

# WORK HARD – PLAY HARD

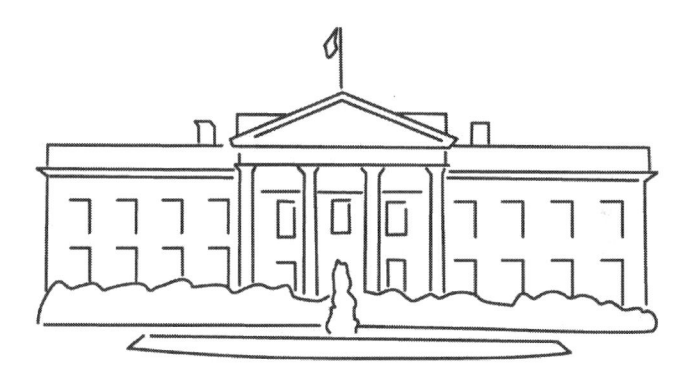

Things returned to normal when I got back from the FDA debacle in Maryland. I was disillusioned but I carried on. I had to keep my focus. I went back to teaching (which I loved) and finger pricking 12-16 times a day (which I hated). There would be no Diasensor in my life and I would have to draw blood forever.

One day after school the phone rang. It was a call from Biocontrol Technology. They asked if I would like to move to Pittsburgh and work for their company. I had enjoyed my time in Pittsburgh as a student at Duquesne, but I explained that I loved Florida and despised cold weather. I was also a devoted Broward County teacher working toward becoming an administrator. They sweetened the deal by offering a job during the summer with a great salary plus housing and a car. I wanted to speak to my husband first, but I promised to call them back.

Larry and I talked it over and his biggest concern was my nighttime blood sugar lows. I had those for years until I went gluten and grain free in 2009. We put together a plan that I would call the front desk and have three wake up calls per night <u>and</u> I would also use an alarm. We told the front desk that if I didn't answer they had permission to enter, (if they knocked and I still didn't answer). Can you imagine waking up three times per night to check blood sugar levels? That was my reality for years.

**Gail's Rule Number Ten:** If you are a diabetic, take precautions when traveling alone. Make sure everyone is aware that you have this disease. Set up calls from the front desk if you are at a hotel, and use an alarm.

With iPhones, setting an alarm is easy now. I still wake myself up occasionally if I travel alone. Old habits die hard. Once that issue was covered we talked about the kids and decided together that if I could help get this technology approved by the FDA, I should do it. Larry would be in charge of the kids. So off I went to Pittsburg to try to make a difference.

While there, I found a new respect for people who put themselves in medical studies and research. Medical research is amazing and intriguing, but very difficult. I spent weeks hooked up to the Diasensor. The only fun thing about being hooked up to the blood machine was the "no finger pricking." I could give my fingers a break, but I couldn't eat because they gave me sugar through an IV.

It was an exciting endeavor. For a moment in time, again, I thought Biocontrol could get FDA approval. The technology never made it to the market, so we know how that story ended. Big Pharma with their deep pockets and far reaching tentacles swept this machine under the rug, never to be heard from again. I know it worked, because I used it, but it didn't matter then, and it doesn't matter now. While I put my life on the line with many other people, including diabetic teenagers, to test the device, the political wheel did away with any product that could hurt the testing companies who make millions on those blood-collecting strips.

**Gail's Rule Number Eleven:** If you are a diabetic and need a new blood testing machine because the one you are using is malfunctioning, call the company and tell them you want a free machine. You should be able to get it because the money is not in the machine; it's in the strips.

During those three months in Pittsburgh, I had been a willing test dummy. My blood sugars were lowered down to 30 and up to 900 in order to get the information that was needed to help my fellow diabetics and me. The end result was back to finger pricking 15+ times per day with no real end in sight.

Despite the outcome, I did it because I cared and because Fred Cooper, the head of Biocontrol, was a great leader. He also cared - deeply. He valued my contribution to the research. He wanted me to educate the public. He created a positive company culture. He thought everyone should have some type of fun in their work lives, even though what we were doing was serious. Company staff would go out every Friday and socialize. What happened to Fred after the Diasensor was stopped is a disgrace. He lost everything, and he didn't deserve it. The bad guys won again.

My last two weeks in Pittsburgh I decided I wanted to start calling the White House so I could try to see then-Vice President Al Gore. I was told I needed a reason to see Al Gore. I said I had a reason. The rise in diabetes in the US was going to elevate it to epidemic. The complications were going to cost the country billions. The person on the other end of the line asked where I was from. I explained that I was from Florida but was in Pittsburgh testing out a product to save lives. A week later there were bets around the office about whether I would get in or not. Everyone bet against me except Fred and the doctor running the study, Dr. Fine!

A week later, I got an invitation to the White House from Al Gore. I was allowed to walk through the halls of the Senate and Congressional offices and speak to representatives. When asked if I was a democrat or a republican, I explained that I am a diabetic American and that's what is important. Political party shouldn't matter when dealing with issues of health.

When I finally got to the White House and spoke to one of Vice President Gore's aides, Toby Donenfeld, I noticed her hands were shaking. I told her she was having low blood sugar. She asked what it was. I gave her a snack and she became an intent listener. I spoke to Toby about the Diasensor, and what I was trying to do. I spoke about Pittsburgh and my experience with the FDA. I stressed how important it was for diabetic Americans to have access to this machine. I laid out my case. She asked if I would be willing to write a newsletter and work with Al Gore if he were elected President. I agreed. As we know, Al Gore did not win the election, and although I got a VIP tour and spoke to various congressmen, my time and trouble were wasted. Biocontrol and Fred Cooper were destroyed and everything was swept under the rug. The legacy of the FDA with regard to diabetics in America is: a disease and its complications reaching epidemic proportions.

# 10

# WHEN LIFE DEALS YOU A BAD HAND, GO AHEAD AND PLAY IT

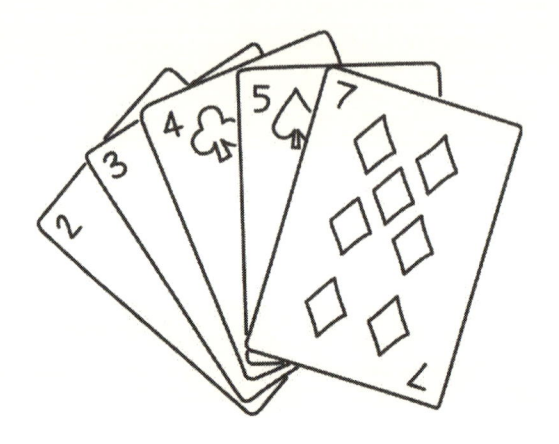

The events that took place after the FDA and my Pittsburgh summer were turning points in the history of my health that shook me even more than dealing with diabetes. Out of nowhere I seemed to be getting really sick again and I didn't know why.

My diabetes was strictly controlled. I continued the protocol of taking multiple shots a day using my Medi-Jector and pricking my poor battered fingers. My biggest fear was never a blood sugar low but instead a high. My HbA1c (glycohemoglobin – which is used to diagnose diabetes) amazed doctors because it was always in the 4's and 5's. Anything below 5.7 is considered normal. It didn't make me nervous to have a really low reading. I would rather die in my sleep from a blood sugar crash than die without all my body parts.

At this point in the 90s, my diabetes was not the problem. Instead, I had other horrible symptoms. I began to bleed from my eyes. I couldn't breath and I was becoming increasingly exhausted. At one point, I exited my school in an ambulance. I discovered that I was having a reaction to the toxic mold in my classroom and all the portables I taught in. It was bad enough to know that the teachers at my school were exposed to asbestos, but who knew about the mold back then? That mold was killing me and I became disabled. I went from an active, vibrant, and somewhat healthy person to a completely sick person. I had handled almost everything like a champ, but at this point I was emotionally spent dealing with health issues. For a while I felt like it was game over and I went home to die.

But my depression didn't last long. I couldn't accept that I had put so much energy into staying on top of my diabetes, only to die of some mystery disease. I rallied and embarked on a new journey. I was going to find out what in heaven (or hell) was going on in my body. By the time all the doctors were done my diagnoses were: chronic fatigue syndrome, fibromyalgia, asthma, vitiligo (loss of pigment – my skin turned from olive to lily white), carpal tunnel syndrome in both wrists, arthritis in my back, full blown osteoporosis, Hashimoto's, severe allergies to my environment, mold allergies, food allergies, and finally, alopecia (hair loss). I was taking 39 prescription medications. Once my hair began falling out in clumps and I ended up with a huge bald spot, I started asking the questions I needed answered.

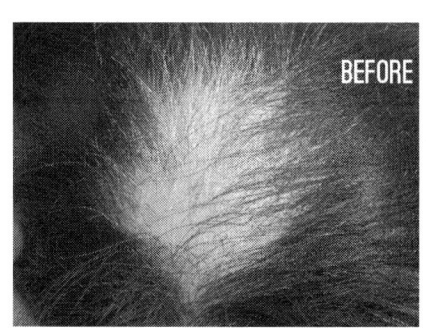

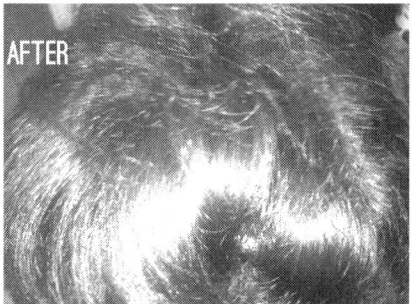

BEFORE AFTER

I never thought I'd say this, but I am grateful that my hair fell out. It saved my life, Lannie's life, and even Larry benefited from my alopecia. At the time, I wasn't able to see the silver lining. I just knew I had to fix it and I had work to do. I took out my computer and started on a new quest for knowledge.

I sought out a dermatologist to deal with my alopecia immediately. My first pick was a bust. Her exact words were, "Oh, you have alopecia, no biggy!" No discussion on treatment, no discussion on what it was or why it was happening to me. I wonder if she would think it was "no biggy" if she went bald? She was the worst. I never went back to her.

My hair loss propelled me into full-blown research mode. You would have thought all the other autoimmune diseases I came down with would have triggered that response, but they didn't. I just couldn't live without my hair. I would sometimes look up at the sky and say, "Hey, you up there! I refuse to go out of this world the way I came into it, white and bald." I wasn't sure anyone was up there, but I said it anyway.

It was too late to do anything about the vitiligo. I had lost all my pigment and was ghostly white, but I was going to stop the balding at all costs. Vanity is a ruthless taskmaster! I could barely get out of bed, but I forged ahead.

It's hard to fix something when you don't know exactly what is broken, so I started my research with general search terms. "WHAT IS CAUSING MY BODY TO GO HAYWIRE?"I wanted to delve into the "why" of diseases. Why me? Why this? What genes make people like my sister and me sick? I was hoping that I would follow a path that would lead to the "why this happened" instead of the treatment.

Simultaneously, I was looking for a doctor with a brain and some knowledge about nutrition, who might be able to help save my hair. I finally found one, Dr. Janee Steinberg. When I walked into her office she said, "Oh, alopecia," and asked her nurse to come in and hold my hand while she shot cortisone into my scalp. That battle went on for quite a long time, and the real research to save my life began.

Sadly, Dr. Steinberg passed away. But I still need to thank her. She treated me with compassion and competence, but lost her own life to cancer in 2012. Thank you Dr. Steinberg. You were the very best in your field. Thank you for keeping my hair on my head while I learned how to do it without medication.

***Gail's Rule Number Twelve:*** Research doctors on Vitals (https://www.vitals.com) and Health Grades (https://www.healthgrades.com). Make sure you put as much time into finding a great doctor as you do when shopping for a car – more on this later. If it's something really important always get two opinions and when they both differ, go for a third. Once that is done always research new ways to treat the same diseases. You'll be surprised what you find out. Doctors don't always know what is new on the horizon or if there is a healthier option without the nasty drugs. Don't be afraid to share your information with the doctor of your choice. I'll say it again. Own your health and educate yourself.

# 11

## 2009- GLUTEN FREE GAIL IS BORN

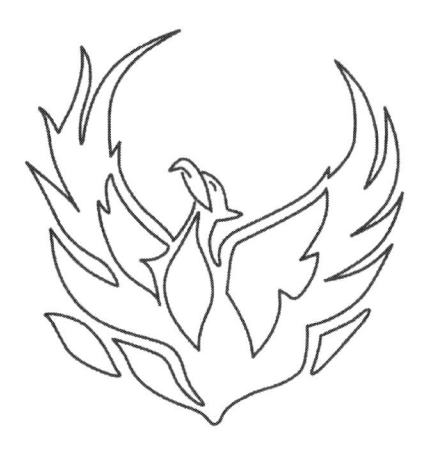

I remember sitting in my endocrinologist's office at age 59 in tears.

"Dr. Carrington, why am I getting disease after disease, even with my healthy lifestyle? I exercise, eat right, religiously monitor my blood sugar levels....why???"

I begged him not to give me any more crap about polyglandular failure. And then he said it again.

"You have polyglandular failure."

I went nuts and screamed, "but WHY????"

Polyglandular failure is a fancy medical term for Shit Outta Luck. My body was continuously breaking down and my immune system was in overdrive, attacking my body. Autoimmune diseases are skyrocketing today and again my question, and yours, should be "why?"

Doctors need to stop offering more drugs to "treat" these conditions and focus on finding the root cause. Some of the drugs they offer are worse than the disease. It's an old joke by now that listening to the Big Pharma television commercials is terrifying as they list the side effects of these drugs that are supposed to help. The list is enough to scare anyone.

***Gail's Rule Number Thirteen:*** If you don't like the answers you get from a physician and deep down in your gut you know something isn't right, do your own homework!

When I left Dr. Carrington's office I had one thing on my mind. I was going to get answers. I was not taking another chemical treatment, medication, or more cortisone-filled needles in my poor scalp. I was going to get answers and fix my body. I didn't really know if I could but I was going to try.

My first goal was to understand the human body and the process that my body went through before an autoimmune disease struck. The next goal was to understand genetics and the role it played in my health. Only 10% of disease stems from genes the other 90% is environment and stress. Finally the most important lesson was about what caused our genes to start the war in our bodies and continue the attack. This is where I read research from Europe about gluten and what it did to the human body, and not just my human body. This was the jackpot. I found the common denominator, the culprit, if you will. Gluten.

So now with all this information in my hands I analyzed my research. Stress was the first part. I realized that being pregnant is a huge stress on the body. When my sister was murdered during my first pregnancy, the stress was catastrophic. Genetics was the second part and I had the genes for autoimmune diseases. Environment was another part and I discovered that my environment was toxic (as is everyone's which is why I wrote this book). Stir that all together in a pot and you've got a toxic stew.

My brain couldn't even wrap itself around what I was reading. I spent three days sitting at my computer reading research paper after research paper. I wondered why the hell my endocrinologist knew nothing about celiac disease or problems with this stuff called gluten. Why weren't people in our country being warned about WHEAT, a very bad GMO with toxic chemicals sprayed on it to make it grow faster and bigger to feed the world and make money, at the expense of our health? We were all eating something that started with two chromosomes and now had eight.

Once I had these facts I set out to find out where this gluten stuff was hiding. This was 2009 and <u>nothing</u> about gluten was being talked about. Finding what to eat was going to be a challenge to say the least. I had to go from eating all those supposedly healthy grains as a vegetarian to eating meat. I had also become allergic to things like eggs, dairy, nuts (but not all nuts), string beans, trout, etc. This was going to take time and it was going to spread beyond food and into every aspect of my life. I would need to find toothpaste and floss without gluten. My life, again, was going to change completely. I was exhausted but interested to discover if gluten free was the answer.

I quickly turned my kitchen into a gluten-free facility. Larry, who is always my support system, decided it was safer for him to go gluten free as well to avoid cross contamination. My crockpot sat on my counter and I bought my first bread machine. Game on. *Within the first week of going gluten free, my hair stopped falling out!* I broke down in tears. I had actually stopped the progression of one of my diseases. I was on to something. At that point, I wasn't sure what gluten free was going to do for my other autoimmune diseases.

I called Lannie one week after I began my gluten-free diet and explained what I was doing. I told her she needed to do it with me because we always did things together. Together we waged war on the American diet. As I sit and write I am crying again. We turned many of our diseases around. My autoimmune diseases are not gone (they will never be gone), but most are in complete remission. I have a full head of hair on my head and I am dancing regularly. I am out of bed and my chronic fatigue/fibromyalgia are a thing of the past. I take two medications now instead of 39. I take insulin and a compounding thyroid medication. I only take four to eight shots of insulin a day and not thirteen to control my disease. I am no longer a brittle type 1. The compounding thyroid medication is a low dosage and free of all Big Pharma byproducts, gluten, and chemicals. I have my T3 compounded without any colors or chemicals.

In the second half of this book, I urge you to detox. We all have to. Poisons are everywhere but the trick is to know where they lurk and get rid of as many as possible. Visit the Environmental Working Group (ewg.org) website as well as the Silent Spring Institute website (silentspring.org). Order a "Detox Me Action Kit" and discover how many toxins are present in your blood stream. The number may alarm you. Download the Detox Me app and get educated. Go gluten free and see how it makes you feel. Investigate, take action, and spread the word. Help your children stay healthy before they develop our modern diseases. Let this book be your starting point.

## 12

# IT'S NEVER TOO LATE

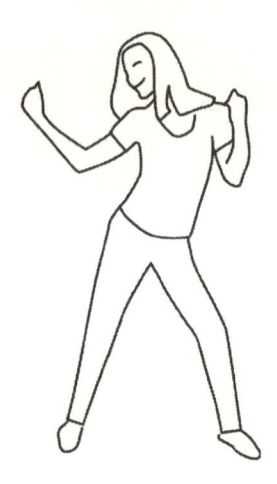

I am a survivor and that is what I have discovered by writing this book. I survived physical, mental, emotional, and sexual abuse all before the age of 14. What happened to me as a child made me strong enough to handle all of the adversity I encountered as an adult. But my coping skills and my motivators prevented me from becoming a <u>healthy</u> adult. I used anger, fear, and perfectionism to drive me, and that is how I got sick. I wonder what would have happened to me if I had not suffered all that abuse? Would my journey have been different? Would I have made different choices? I can't say for sure, but it begs reflection. Today I understand what makes a healthy body. It's a healthy mind.

I did all the right things with regard to my physical health. I ate right, exercised, and was an advocate for myself and others. I took a proactive attitude toward everything. But my mind still wasn't healed. I wasn't happy and I needed professional help.

I joke and say I have always felt nuts, but I never really thought about going for real professional counseling until these last few years – well after the age of 65. Even though I'm at the end of my life, I decided it was worth it to seek help for all the damage that had been done to me. My psychiatrist gave me homework. I had to pick three affirmations to say to myself each day. I picked:

*I matter and what I have to say matters*
*I forgive myself for not being perfect*
*I am healthy*

I say these every day. At first I laughed out loud. But now, I've been saying them long enough that I'm starting to believe them!

Seeking professional help and joining a 12-step program forced me to take stock. I had lived most of my life in fear. As a child I was afraid of everything, and as an adult those fears have manifested as different phobias like: fear of flying, fear of getting on a cruise, fear of traveling in a car. I do these things, but I'm always afraid. I fear other people and trust very few. I had dozens of years fueled by fear, anger, and hate.

I had to commit to fixing my head. I walked out of my first 12-step program ten years ago because I couldn't handle the "God" talk. I wasn't a believer. I lost all faith during my childhood. But my son suggested another 12-step program, so five years ago I committed to giving it another try.

In this program, the most important thing you learn is to respond instead of react. Your cortisol kicks in if you sweat the small stuff all the time, and the mind-body connection gets frazzled. You learn to say no. You learn you can't fix others. You are powerless over absolutely everyone, and you use journaling to acknowledge and record this powerlessness. You learn gratitude and positive thinking. You use meditation and breath work. But you are allowed to feel the hurt and pain and you are allowed to have the anger and cry the tears. You don't have to hide the bad stuff anymore. The pain of my childhood and my sister's murder had been buried so deeply I couldn't heal. I believe it caused my diseases.

If you're interested in a 12-step program, but the first one you attend doesn't work for you, don't give up. Keep going and keep trying until you find a group that resonates with you. I found mine and it changed my life. I was not only able to accept myself, even though I'm not perfect, but I was able to better understand those closest to me as well. My husband Larry had a terrible upbringing too and it has left scars. Those around you are carrying heavy burdens and understanding that helps understand them. You will make mistakes of course and you'll have bad days, but if you put in the work, you'll get better. You'll start to find balance. You'll be more emotionally available and learn to productively communicate how you feel.

It has taken time but I'm out of denial and able to express myself now.

The walls I built are coming down, brick by brick. I'm letting others in, really in. I'm now grateful for who I am and what I've become. I'm strong and resilient. I'm smart and a lifelong lover of learning. When I'm down, I'm never down for long. I've forgiven everyone – my mother for her cruelty, my father for abandoning me, Janice for succumbing to addiction, anyone who hurt me. I am a stubborn survivor, but healthier now than I've ever been in mind and spirit. I've exorcised my demons. My journey was horrible but I made it and I'm excited to help others.

Each day I work on learning something new about who I am and who I was. I live each day to the fullest. I am excited for tomorrow. My son Jonathan was right and I'm grateful that he urged me to try a 12-step one more time.

But just as the physical journey is ongoing, the mental journey is too. When I decided to get certified to teach ZUMBA®, I was afraid. What would my students think of me? Would they think I was fat? Would they think I shouldn't teach dance at all? When I thought about publishing this book, I had to face my fears again. What would people think when they discovered so much about my life? Would anyone find the information I was offering useful? I still struggle but now I have the right coping mechanisms. It's never too late.

**_Gail's Final Rules_**: Don't dwell on looking backwards. Always look ahead. Drop the anger. It'll make you sick. Don't fill your brain with garbage. Find forgiveness for those who have hurt or damaged you. Don't think you know everything because if you do, you'll be closed off to learning. Stress is a killer. How you handle it makes all the difference. Don't be reactive. Be calm and take deep breaths.

## 13

## BREAKING UP IS HARD TO DO

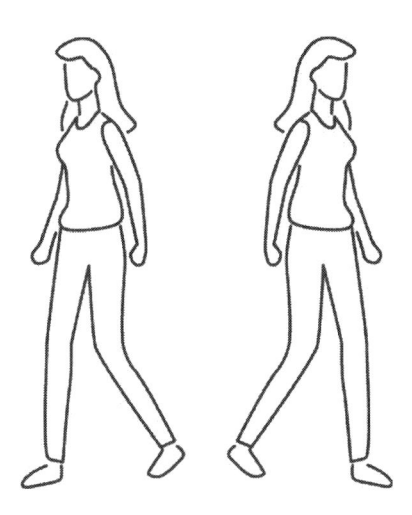

Before I launch into the discoveries I've made over the years regarding food and environment, I want to return to the issue of finding a good doctor. It seems to me that people just go to any doctor without giving it real thought. As a matter of fact if people would put as much energy into finding a reputable doctor as they do when buying a car, lives would be healthier and less people would be placed on medication as a first line of defense. How to find the best doctor should be on everyone's to-do list whenever an issue comes up.

First of all, own your diseases and do not rely on the medical professionals to do it. I know I keep saying it, but it's true. All doctors, whether good or bad, are going to miss important information with your health because they are truly overworked. Look at the medical offices and wait-times to get an appointment, see a doctor, or get a blood test. Why would anyone think a medical professional is really going to take a thorough look at blood tests?

With me a fiasco occurred recently when I didn't pay attention to one test because I was so busy. I started feeling really weird and began my education again. What could cause pain all over and not be fibromyalgia or was I finally having a reoccurrence of my fibromyalgia after years in remission? I couldn't understand why this would be happening now. This pain seemed different, not quite like the fibromyalgia, but the confusion was over how tired I was. I guess it didn't really matter why. Here I was again gathering up my blood tests while I did my research, and right there on my second blood test was my answer. Sadly none of my really good doctors picked up my low ferritin because the test read "green," as in normal.

So what is normal? A ferritin level of 26 is normal on my test, but 26 is anything but normal. On my Quest test 26 was one point away from being abnormal. I thought both doctors had missed it until I went to my new thyroid doctor who immediately looked at my blood work and said that I needed to be on an iron pill because my ferritin was so low. I asked why he had not recommended it until now? I found out that my other doctor's office, where the test had been taken, had never faxed those results nor had they faxed my thyroid information. I had sent the office the fax number and a note to be sure to send all my results to two doctors, but they just didn't do it. It wasn't intentional, but it was careless. This is why you, the patient, need to stay on top of these things.

My doctor recommended what I was already doing. I had put myself on three iron pills a day until I could get my blood into the 50-100 range. Looking at my "normal" 26 was making me sick and if I had not seen it myself and began taking something for low ferritin, I was going to get really sick and the pain in my body was only going to get worse. I was using up all my stored iron. That is what a low ferritin means. Since my family has a history of bone cancer along with iron deficiency anemia with the autoimmune disease called Intrinsic B, these are the kinds of tests that need to be watched. I had hoped that all my doctors had looked at these things but I was wrong.

The reason for this chapter is right here! If I had not looked at my blood work from Quest, read my results, understood my results, then handed that test information to my doctor to discuss, I would have been in a hospital in a few weeks and a great deal of money would have been spent on one stupid missed blood test.

I also needed to find out <u>why</u> my iron count was going low. The answer for that could be how much iron I ingest which is probably too little. I had been creeping into the no-meat zone again in my diet and this was the result. See what I mean about forgetting what I already know? If I don't eat meat or certain foods where was my iron going to come from? So I went back to eating some grass-fed organic meat twice a week. You would think by now I would remember these things but even I need to re-read my own book!

## My Ferritin Fix

In addition to adding grass-fed beef to my diet, I upped my magnesium citrate to 500 mg's a day and began taking two pills in the morning and one at night. I removed foods I thought might be inflammatory by taking my MRT test again (see recommended testing below). The test showed that sweet potatoes where highly reactive so I stopped eating them. I upped my T3 with the guidance of my doctor and within two weeks I was not longer hurting, my weight was finally going down, I was sleeping without pain all over my body, and off I went to dance. Life was good again.

Like so many aspects of a lifestyle change, it does take work to understand blood tests and your own body, but it is worth it. The only thing I needed some guidance with was my thyroid pill, because adjustments need to be made to that over time. I am still dealing with thyroid issues in 2019, but because of what I have done over the years, I am able to isolate problems quickly and focus on targeted solutions. That is the best thing about my journey and my conscientiousness. I always know when something is amiss. I find someone who understands my goals and we work together to heal me without chemicals and prescriptions. I have no choice but to take thyroid medication, but again, I use a compounding pharmacy and my pills are made with rice powder.

I recently read an article in the newspaper that said many doctors are unable to read your blood tests. This is no surprise to me as the doctors I have seen in the past have missed my celiac disease, my diabetes, my autoimmune rash, misdiagnosed my B12 deficiency, and most recently missed my low ferritin. It's important that every patient get a copy of their blood results and learn how to read them. When something says abnormal, ask the doctor what that means regarding a particular test. Sometimes it means nothing. Sometimes it means everything. If you have a disease, it is your disease, not the doctor's.

Make sure you are registered with Quest or LabCorp. If you do this they will send you your test results and you can keep them in your hands and go over them with your doctor when you have an office visit. If you are unable to read them, use your computer to find explanations for what each test means. Study and learn how to read these results so you can have an intelligent discussion about them with your physician.

For instance, if you know that your HbA1c is too high, you have to address it at the doctor. If you don't get this test done regularly, I suggest you start doing so. This test checks the average of your blood sugars for three months. It explains how your body is using insulin or not using insulin. Type 2 diabetes is so out of control today due to the unhealthy American diet, that everyone should be aware of that HbA1c blood test. If you have diabetes, it will be discovered early with regular testing, and you can start adjusting your life to avoid its many complications.

All of this is part of taking ownership of our health and the advocacy we need to practice on our own behalf. Gut instinct, research, and experience will yield the best results when finding a doctor. And if you have to break up with your doctor, do it, even if breaking up is hard to do.

Now let me discuss how seriously I take choosing a good doctor or hospital. This is where buying a car comes into play for me. When I need to get a new car, I get out a notebook and begin reading about cars I think I like. I read consumer reviews and safety reports. With as much information in hand as possible, I head to the dealership and ask to test drive my top candidates. Which car has the best drive and road feel? Which car is the roomiest? Which car can I see out of on all sides? Which car is highly rated by consumers?

Do that when looking for a medical professional. It will make all the difference to your health and well-being. Here are some of my most trusted resources and I use all of them during a search. I don't just rely on one.

*www.Vitals.com:* Find, rate, or check up on a doctor in the United States. Search by location, specialty, or ailment.

*www.HealthGrades.com*: Find a doctor, view background information, write a doctor review. Types: All Specialties.

*www.SurgeonRatings.org*: Contains data on more than four million major surgeries and 50,000 doctors who performed them.

*www.FSMB.org:* Federation of State Medical Boards is a national not-for-profit organization representing the 70 medical and osteopathic boards of the United States.

*www.CertificationMatters.org:* Certification Matters is a patient-friendly website of the American Board of Medical Specialties (ABMS) that allows patients to check for free if their doctor is Board Certified by an ABMS.

When you look for a good doctor look at their state credentials, see if they have had any reprimands or loss of a license like I did with Randall Hrabko, M.D. of California. He lost his license at least four times, was involved in the death of a young girl (my sister), gave a woman herpes and lost his case, and yet kept moving and getting a new license. He is still in practice with a 3.3 out of 5 rating on Vitals and 5-star rating on Health Grades. All the bad information went away and now he looks great. Would you want to use this type of doctor? I would not. Here is where certification information is more helpful. Bad information goes away after so many years and you can never find out unless you are relentless with your research.

I want to understand into whose hands I am about to put my health. I act as if it is a life or death choice, which it can be. What is so sad today is that hospitals accept the fact that doctors are going to make mistakes and kill people by accident. I would rather choose my own doctor, but even with the best, mistakes can happen. Choosing wisely in conjunction with understanding blood work equals a greater chance of success. I can now interpret <u>all</u> of my blood tests and Lannie is even better at it. That was a lot of learning! Approximately 3500 people died in 2017 at the hands of their doctors. Why not take the time and look for the best to mitigate risk?

When my gallbladder started to fail I went to three doctors and interviewed each one. These doctors had five star ratings and the correct certifications without any malpractice issues. I picked the one I thought I had the best rapport with. My instinct was correct. I loved him. I needed to feel trust with someone who was going to cut into me! This was my very first surgery. I recommended him to someone else, and they also loved him. Taking this process seriously is necessary to make the best choice when dealing with medical issues. It is your life or the life of a loved on hanging in the balance.

**Testing**

This section is very important as a companion to your doctor search because without the right tests, it is impossible to know exactly what is going on inside our bodies. The regular blood panels done at the doctor's office are incomplete and unless you ask for some of these tests, you won't get them. It took me years to learn exactly what I needed in order to get an overall picture of my health. The tests I mention on this page I have found to be the most accurate and reliable health benchmarks. If you can, learn how to interpret the results of these tests as well.

### *SpectraCell*
https://www.spectracell.com/patients/patient-micronutrient-testing/
Micronutrient testing

### *Oxford Biomedical Technologies*
http://nowleap.com/the-patented-mediator-release-test-mrt/
This food intolerance testing is the best on the market. Following the results will completely change the way you eat and how you feel

### *Cologuard*
https://www.cologuardtest.com/
Colon cancer testing at home - available only by prescription

***Genova***
https://www.gdx.net/product/gut-immunology-test-stool
Gut immunology tests and more

***Ferritin Testing***
https://www.mayoclinic.org/tests-procedures/ferritin-test/about/pac-20384928
Ferritin testing is important because it indicates whether the body is storing too much or too little iron

***Methylmalonic Acid***
https://www.healthline.com/health/methylmalonic-acid-test#modal-close
This test determines the correct B12 storage levels

***CMP - Comprehensive Metabolic Panel***
https://www.urmc.rochester.edu/encyclopedia/content.aspx?contenttypeid=167&contentid=comprehensive_metabolic_panel
This checks basic bodily functions and can be done at a blood lab by prescription

***CBC with Differential Screening (Complete Blood Count)***
http://www.healthcheckusa.com/blood-type-count/complete-blood-count-cbc-with-differential.aspx
This tests for various disease states such as anemia, leukemia, inflammation, among others

***HbA1c (Hemoglobin A1c)***
https://www.mayomedicallaboratories.com/test-catalog/Clinical+and+Interpretive/82080
This is the correct test for diabetes

***Vitamin D Blood Test***
https://www.vitamindcouncil.org/about-vitamin-d/testing-for-vitamin-d/
You want it above 40 but preferably around 70

***Autoimmune Panel***
This test is important if you know something is wrong but can't get a diagnosis

***HLA Typing (Human Leukocyte Antigen)***

https://www.sciencedirect.com/topics/medicine-and-dentistry/human-leukocyte-antigen
This is for celiac disease and other immune diseases

### Heavy Metal Testing
https://bengreenfieldfitness.com/podcast/biohacking-podcasts/the-crucial-dos-and-donts-of-heavy-metal-testing-and-metal-detoxification/
Blood and/or Urine

### Stool Testing
https://www.gdx.net/product/comprehensive-digestive-stool-analysis-cdsa
For H. pylori bacteria and other bacterial infections

### Ova and Parasite testing
https://www.healthline.com/health/stool-ova-parasites-test

### Lyme Disease testing
https://www.cdc.gov/lyme/diagnosistesting/index.html

### Epstein-Barr Virus Antibody Panel
https://www.healthline.com/health/epstein-barr-virus-test

### Cytomegalovirus Panel
https://www.news-medical.net/health/What-is-Cytomegalovirus.aspx

### Microalbum Urine Test
https://www.mayoclinic.org/tests-procedures/microalbumin/about/pac-20384640

### Cardio IQ Advanced Lipid Panel
http://www.tfmhealth.com/cardio-iq—-what-is-tested.html

### Thyroid Testing
http://www.healthcheckusa.com/thyroid-tests/panels/complete-thyroid-function-panel.aspx
Must be complete and include thyroid antibodies

### Lifeline Screening
http://www.lifelinescreening.com/
This test is preventative but well worth it. It can detect heart disease, osteoporosis, and cancer early.

### *Breast Thermography*
http://www.breastthermography.com/

Thermography can detect cancer years before it manifests. In Fort Lauderdale, I use a clinic called www.ThermographyFirst.com and found their care excellent.

Now it's time to expose toxic America. I cannot write about everything in our world that is toxic, so it is up to the next generation to do their homework and fight big corporations. Our food is toxic, our beds are toxic, our clothes are toxic, and our world is becoming more and more toxic every day. Can we fix it? I don't know anymore. I am sad for what we have done to this beautiful world but if you do something in your own home like replacing plastic bottles with re-usable, that alone will help the fish in the oceans and the oceans themselves. Commit to starting somewhere. I hope this book opens your eyes and your heart and I hope it inspires you to take action. Are you ready?

… PART II: ARE YOU READY TO DETOX?

UNDERSTANDING WHAT'S IN YOUR EVERYDAY FOODS

# 14

# A1 VS A2 COWS AND THE BENEFITS OF RAW MILK

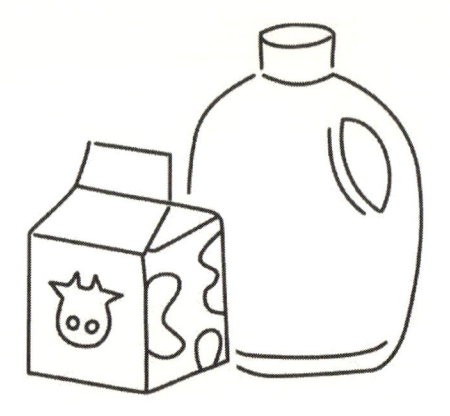

Did you know that there are two kinds of cows? I didn't. It was only when I started to get sick that I began to investigate <u>everything</u> I ate and <u>everything</u> I touched. I never imagined that I would be finding out that our cows produce unhealthy dairy. The kinds of milk I had been drinking and the cheese I had been eating had been making my hair fall out and cause other health concerns. So I did what I thought was smart and stopped drinking milk and eating cheese.

Once I stopped eating cheese and drinking milk, I began to deal with osteoporosis due to a lack of calcium and enzymes that I needed to keep my bones healthy, so once again I was prompted by real life circumstances to continue my research. I always start with a question or questions. Could I find something to replace what I call the "dead food" found in the grocery stores? Were there any "real" cows left? Could those cows make me milk?

It is now more than a decade later and the answer is yes! I drink milk and eat cheese, just not the kind of milk and cheese most Americans drink and eat. What you find in the store are dead and over-processed dairy products. I eat only raw dairy from A2 cows that produce the necessary enzymes and good bacteria that I need to keep my gut healthy. You probably want to know why anyone would care about the different numbers of the cows and why cows would be assigned numbers. I asked myself the same questions. And I studied to understand the difference. We should all want the A2 cows and this is why.

Let's start with the names of the cows that are the "real thing." I began to look for Jersey and Guernsey cows that produce the A2 milk. Any cow claiming to be A2 must go through rigid testing. When I first started the switch, I would ask for certification information on the cows so I could review the requirements and familiarize myself with the certification process. What I didn't want then and don't want now are the A1 cows whose family genetics have been altered into something not so healthy. These cows are Holsteins, they are black and white and produce something quite different than the non-genetically-modified cows. What the black and white cows produce can make us sick and helped cause my multiple autoimmune diseases. What could they be doing to your health?

I did more research to find out how it all went down. Many moons ago we only had A2 cows that produced a healthy dose of live enzymes helpful to the human body. For some reason, a mutation occurred, and the A1 cow was "born." The A1 mutation caused the BCM7 (Beta-casamorphin-7) peptide to appear in A1 cow's milk (or the protein found in cow's milk which is casein). BCM7 has narcotic side effects and has been known to cause lactose intolerance. So not only is it bad for you, it's also addictive. No wonder it's so hard to give up cheese! But the A1 cows produced more milk and the farmers could get rich. Sound familiar?

Remember when I said that I got an autoimmune disease from drinking A1 cow's milk? Well, there is research that says A1 cow's milk can be linked to type 1 diabetes, allergies, gut problems, and skin conditions. I decided to put the research aside and just make a switch to A2 to see what would happen.

The rest is history. I eat raw dairy every three days because I rotate my foods, and to my surprise, I don't get sick from it anymore. Was it because I went to raw dairy or because I went to A2 raw dairy? I can't say for sure. Everyone has to make his or her own decision. I only know that I can now eat cheese and milk from both cows and goats. I am still on the look out for camel's milk because camels and goats only produce A2 proteins and enzymes.

If you have trouble finding good raw milk, look online for local farmers who have A2 cows and buy from them or just stick to all goat milk products and buy raw for the health benefits. This is what I do and I am healthier at 70 than I was at 48. My gut is healed, I am no longer allergic, and my bones are strong. It's a win-win!

Further Reading

If you are reading the paperback instead of the ebook - you can type each title below in your computer search bar and find the referenced article.

A1 Vs. A2 Milk: Does It Matter?

California Dairy Research Foundation A2 Milk Facts

Milk Intolerant? Lactose Might Not Be The Problem

What Is A2 Milk?

## 15

## BPA AND BPAF – DON'T TOUCH THE RECEIPTS

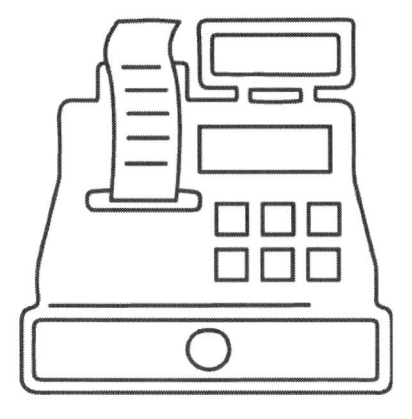

Chemicals lurk everywhere. I knew it would be a tall order to get rid of all of the chemicals that big business was trying to stuff into my small body. But, I could control grabbing receipts when leaving a store or buying products lined with both BPA and BPAF (really bad chemicals).

You might think I'm going overboard and on the verge of paranoia, and I wouldn't disagree. Sometimes I think I am too! But when I read the research on those two chemicals, I decided my new mantra would be, "better nuts than sick." I live by that. I will not get sick again if there is any way to prevent it. I spent too many years feeling miserable and nearly bed ridden, waiting to die. Those days are over for good. So what exactly are BPA and BPAF and what are they doing to my body?

When I want actual facts I go to [PubMed.gov](PubMed.gov) to start an investigation. They have to give you the facts. At least I think they do! In July 2012 they did a study on what this stuff does to our endocrine system and this is where both my sister and I were having problems. BPA mimics the structure and function of estrogen. It can also interact with thyroid hormone and alter its function. If you've ever had hormone issues, you know that any fluctuation in hormone levels can wreak havoc on digestion, weight, energy, fertility, mood, and so much more. Lannie and I both had whacky endocrine systems and I wanted to fix them. I realized I couldn't if I kept grabbing those receipts and then touching my face or eating canned food lined with BPA.

I remember walking into BJ's grocery store one day and while checking out at the register, I met a woman who was wearing gloves. She was the smart one. She knew how bad the receipts were and she didn't want to handle them all day long. I congratulated her and she smiled because she knew that I knew that she wasn't nuts either. Upon returning to the store I saw her again when we happened to land at her checkout line. She wasn't wearing her gloves anymore. I asked her why. She told me that her company would not allow it. The store didn't want her to scare people. She had to choose between losing her job and exposing herself to harmful chemicals daily. She was really upset by that policy. It is a choice no one should have to make.

Why not get the same receipt paper that Whole Foods uses without those chemicals? Of course the culprit is cost. Money will always be more important than the health of our citizens.

So where are these chemicals lurking?
Aluminum Cans have a BPA lining unless they say they don't
ATM Receipts
Lottery tickets
Airline tickets
Cash Register receipts
Prescription labels

Here is what I do to lessen my risk of getting too much of this into my system when it comes to receipts. I make sure that when I purchase something I have them put the toxic receipt into my grocery bag and when I get home I throw it away and wash my hands. I don't even care if they look at me funny. What they think of me is none of my business. What *is* my business is keeping myself and my loved ones healthy.

Canned products also use BPA and BPAF linings. You have to buy only glass products or products that are BPA/BPAF free. I choose to use glass and an added benefit, most glass is still made in America. Some things made here are actually safe. When you purchase glass you make jobs for our citizens and keep people safe at the same time.

Here is my list of cans without BPA linings (also check the Shopping section of this book for other amazing products, all personally vetted by me, so you know they're good)!

***Amy's*** - all of their products. (www.Amys.com)

***American Tuna*** - all of their canned tuna. (www.AmericanTuna.com)

***Annie's Homegrown*** - all of their products are safe. (www.Annies.com)

***Bumble Bee*** - tuna, herring, and sardines canned and produced in the USA. (www.BumbleBee.com)

***Campbell's Soup*** - they started phasing out BPA in 2012 and completed the transition in mid-2017. They replaced the linings with acrylic and polyester alternatives. (www.Campbell.com)

***Crown Prince Naturals*** - I love this natural product - but make sure it is the "Naturals." Check their site for information because it can change every year. More and more of their products are being made without BPAs. (www.CrownPrince.com)

***EarthPure Organic Tomatoes*** - I buy all of their tomato products online. (www.NeilJonesFoodCompany)

***Eden Organics*** – these are my favorites. (www.EdenFoods.com)

***Genova*** - canned tuna only. (www.GenovaSeafood.com)

***Hain Celestial Products*** - they went chemical free in 2014 and I mean <u>all</u> their products. (www.Hain.com)

***Juanitas*** - all canned foods. (www.Juanitas.com)

***Jyoti*** - all of their canned Indian foods. (www.JyotiFoods.com)

***King Oscar Norwegian*** - all of their products. (www.KingOscar.com)

***Muir Glen*** – also one of my favorite companies. All of their products are safe. (www.MuirGlen.com)

***Nature Factor*** - Coconut water. (www.Amazon.com)

***Native Forest*** - another one of my favorites. All of their stuff is chemical-free. (www.EdwardAndSons.com) or (www.ThriveMarket.com)

***Natural Sea*** - a good company that sells tuna, clams and salmon.(www.NaturalSea.com)

## Further Reading

If you are reading the paperback instead of the ebook - you can type each title below in your computer search bar and find the referenced article.

What Is BPA And Why Is It Bad For You?

BPA Replacement Chemical Concern

Mayo Clinic: Nutrition And Healthy Eating

# 16

# BUTTER – THE REAL DEAL

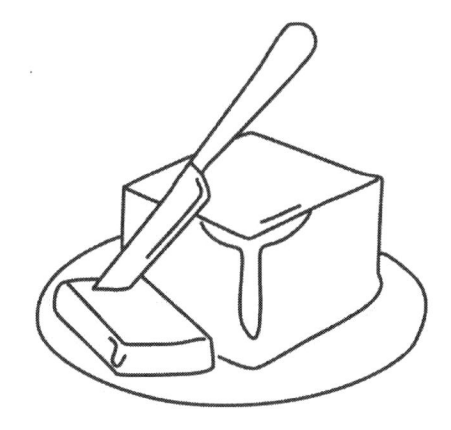

For many years everyone said "real butter" was terrible for our health. I know my mother did and even I did. For a time we told our children that butter was the root of all evil and we got rid of it in our diets. We replaced healthy fats, with fake, unhealthy oils made of ingredients no one can pronounce. Big food companies helped in this unhealthy transition and added insult to injury by putting these concoctions in plastic containers (lined with BPA!). In the early days, we believed that the FDA actually knew what they were doing and the powers that be were looking out for the health of our families. We now know better. So what is wrong with the low fat margarines and butter substitutes that we find in our grocery stores? Why does everyone seem to be buying them?

Marketing is key here of course. It is easy to lie to the public or misinform people with TV commercials and FDA "studies" (invariably industry-funded). Regular folks find it hard to accept that companies and ad agencies have no problem disseminating untruths. They also use a form of brainwashing that involves repeating and showing the same things over and over again – so much so that these things, no matter what they are, are accepted as truth. They also show aspirational images of beautiful, wealthy people eating, drinking, and using what they want to sell. Since most of us aspire to be gorgeous and rich, our brain connects the dots and buys the product. It's not our fault – we're being manipulated.

The truth is, by getting rid of real butter we eliminated butyrate. What the heck is butyrate? I said the same thing, but I didn't say "heck!" Butyrate is a substance that our colon relies on to make energy and our bodies cannot produce enough to keep us healthy. Butyrate puts the healthy bacteria in our gut and without it Americans get sick. My family and I now eat the real thing, and I took it a step further. I actually buy raw butter and take pills that contain this miracle ingredient.

Real butter and cheese are loaded with butyrate. Now comes an unforeseen problem. Our dairy and cows are sick too, so where can we get butyrate if we don't want to consume the butter from this country or cannot consume dairy?

At first I got my butter from Amazon.com. I bought Anchor Butter from New Zealand. New Zealand uses A2 cows that are not toxic and contain Omega 3s, healthy butyrate, and CLAs (a super fatty acid). My local grocery store, Publix, carries cheese from New Zealand, so I used to get cheese there occasionally. But when I really got educated, I began to buy cheese from a farm that sells raw dairy including goat's milk. I recommend this choice above all others, but these alternatives can get expensive.

If you can't afford the New Zealand butter from Amazon, my second choice is Organic Valley, Limited Edition May through September. Use their **_organic_** only in the green colored tin foil. This butter has naturally occurring CLAs and Omega 3s and puts the butyrate back into our diet. I used to buy Organic Valley from time to time but, as I mentioned, I went farm-to-table when I found Marando Farms in Fort Lauderdale. Every Saturday I head there to shop for both local organics and raw dairy. I know many people are afraid of raw, unpasteurized dairy but the truth is that more people get sick and die from the dead dairy in the supermarket. I for one am willing to take my chances with the raw, healthy stuff. So far, it has worked wonders.

### Butyrate and what it can do for the human body:

Butyrate increases the function of our healthy mitochondria. With only unhealthy cells, we all get diseases like I did. These healthy cells are the powerhouses of our body.

Butyrate helps us with physical and metabolic stress.

Butyrate helps control inflammation in our gut which all of us have due to our diets and environment. When the body is in constant inflammation we get diseases.

For those who can't eat dairy, Butyrate can be found in other sources, such as cold potatoes and cold rice. I eat both on occasion since they are gluten free, but they tend to raise my blood sugar, so I have to be very careful. After searching high and low, (so you don't have to), I finally found a pill online made by BodyBio (www.BodyBio.com). I bought Cal-Mag Butyrate. There are other butyrate products that BodyBio makes, so in order to determine which one was the best for me, I asked my doctor and called the company.

I run most of the things I am going to do or take with my favorite doctor who also had to go gluten free with me to get healthy. I know we are always on the same page. I think he is the one who brought up butyrate for my health, and when Dr. Tourgeman suggests, I go out and learn. By the way, when you open the bottle of BodyBio butyrate, it will smell like cheese!

Further Reading

If you are reading the paperback instead of the ebook - you can type each title below in your computer search bar and find the referenced article.

Butyrate: The Surprising Ingredient For Gut And Brain Communication

Butyrate, A Metabolite Of Intestinal Bacteria, Enhances Sleep

What Is Butyrate And Why Should You Care?

# 17

# CANNED TOMATOES – NOT SO HEALTHY

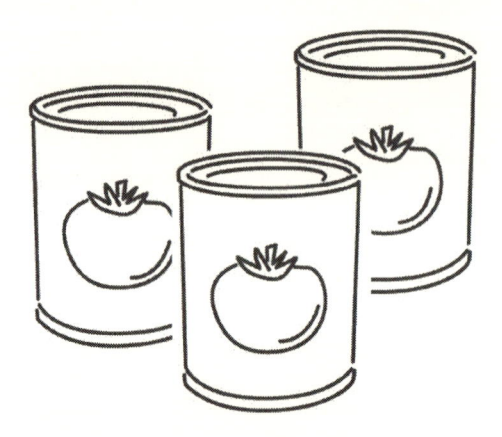

Canned tomatoes are less about the food and more about how they are sold. Of course this assumes you are buying everything organic, which you should! Tomatoes contain a high amount of acid and the cans they use today (see chapter on BPAs) will leach lead into your blood stream.

When I began to learn about canned foods I decided to see what was safe and what I should <u>not</u> buy canned. Later on I learned to buy glass only with certain foods, tomatoes being one of those foods. If people keep eating the kind of canned tomatoes that they sell in the grocery stores, some could die from lead poisoning.

As honest companies began to realize that cheap canning practices were having chemical side effects, they began getting rid of the BPA linings little by little. But tomatoes are so acidic; any chemical replacement will still cause problems. Glass is always the best choice.

Here is what more lead can do to the body, and I said *more* because we already know that there is lead in apple juice, chicken, and now the cans we eat from. Lead affects the brain, can produce heart disease, ups the ante for breast cancer, heightens the risk for prostate cancer, and possibly affects the human reproductive system. Anyone care? Well I did so I started to buy as much as I could in all glass.

And by the way, there are cheap ways to get around the canned tomato problem. Buy organic tomatoes, leave the skin on, throw them in the blender with any spices or salt you might want, and blend. Throw that on your rice or other gluten-free pasta and voila! You have just made homemade tomato sauce. For those of you who want to work harder at it …cook it after blending, and it is more like homemade. The price savings of making your own allows you to purchase organic tomatoes without the side of chemicals seeping from the can. This is good for the environment and good for you.

### *Quick recipe*

Lots of organic tomatoes, salt or no salt, real garlic, oregano, whole real onion and blend. You will be amazed at the results. I know I was when I tried it!

Further Reading

If you are reading the paperback instead of the ebook - you can type each title below in your computer search bar and find the referenced article.

Why You Should Never Use Canned Tomatoes

Fact Or Myth? You Should Never Eat Tomatoes Stored In Cans

One Small Step: Avoiding BPA In Tomatoes

# 18

# CARRAGEENAN – A "HEALTHY" ADDITIVE?

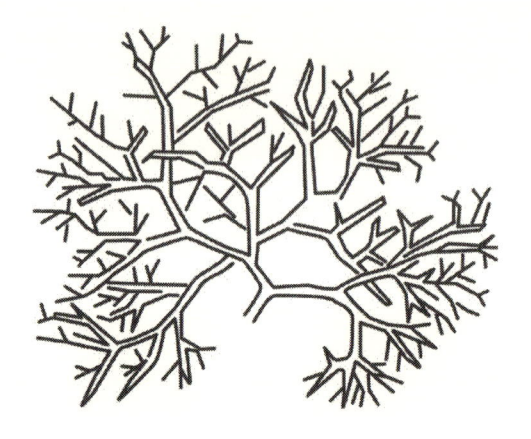

Over the last decade, I've found myself in numerous food predicaments. My body reacts to something negatively and I have to make adjustments or I discover something that urges me to add or subtract items from my diet. During one of these periods, I found myself searching for a calcium source that was not cow's milk or even goat's milk. I wasn't sure if I really needed to get my calcium from dairy, but I thought I would look into nut milks and hemp milk to see what I might find. I went to Whole Foods, pen and paper in hand, and sat on the floor reading labels and taking notes. I wasn't so crazy about the gar gums I saw on various ingredient lists, but what stood out immediately was the carrageenan seaweed. I had no idea what it was and I was seeing more and more of it in healthy foods as well as not so healthy foods. I thought maybe it was a good thing because it was made from seaweed, but being food intolerant, I wanted to know more.

    I didn't buy anything and went home to read about this seaweed product and begin my phone calls. I started that day by calling my son Brett to see if he knew what it was. He is pretty well versed and knowledgeable and I was tired of calling companies. I was hoping he could help. He said, "mom if it is made from seaweed how bad can it be?" I decided to find out more about this mystery ingredient. If you can't spell it, pronounce it, or define it, don't eat it until you know what it is!

I continued calling it the mystery ingredient, yet I was seeing it in more and more foods, including the "healthy" cold cuts in packages that are sold at Whole Foods.

As I came to discover, carrageenan is a nasty chemical hiding in a lot of foods including organic food and most nut milks. It's used as a thickener and fat replacer in processed foods. It has absolutely zero nutritional value as a food additive. I will never eat any food with carrageenan in it, at least not willingly.

Here is the list of some "healthy" products that contain this poison derived from seaweed:

Tofutti milk-free ice cream
YoKids yogurts
Simply Cottage Cheese by Kraft
All nut milks (unless they specifically state "carrageenan free")
Organic creams and milks…but why?
All Applegate Farms cold cuts
Where it can be found elsewhere:
Toothpaste
Gummy products
Dairy
Shoe polish
Shaving cream

It is everywhere. How bad is it? How bad can a thickener be? I mean we use cornstarch to thicken things…not that I eat much corn but this stuff comes from the sea and things from the sea are good. Right? Wrong. It isn't good for the human body.

Dr. Joanne K. Tobacman, MD, Associate Professor of Clinical Medicine at the University of Illinois College of Medicine, a researcher on gut health, has researched the impact that carrageenan has on the human body. Dr. Tobacman said that her research has shown that exposure to carrageenan causes inflammation. When we consume processed foods containing it, we ingest enough to cause inflammation. In 2008 Dr. Tobacman filed a petition with the FDA to asking them to get carrageenan out of the food supply because it was a possible carcinogen. To-date nothing has been done to remove it from our food supply and don't forget the pet food supply as well.

The FDA said that there wasn't enough proof and that no one has clearly died from the use of this product. Well I disagree! If all disease begins with an unhealthy gut and inflammation, then why would we choose to eat something that might break our guts wide open? Not enough proof? We know how I feel about the FDA. For myself, I don't pick that poison. I choose to find products without this word, which by the way I still have trouble spelling and pronouncing. In 2014, the nut milk companies got enough hate mail about seaweed carrageenan to take it out of many of the healthy products. They must know something!

Further Reading

If you are reading the paperback instead of the ebook - you can type each title below in your computer search bar and find the referenced article.

Carrageenan: Carcinogen Allowed In Organic Food?

USDA Decides To Allow Carrageenan In Organic Foods Despite Health Concerns

Is Carrageenan Safe?

# 19

# CHEMICAL WARFARE EVERY DAY

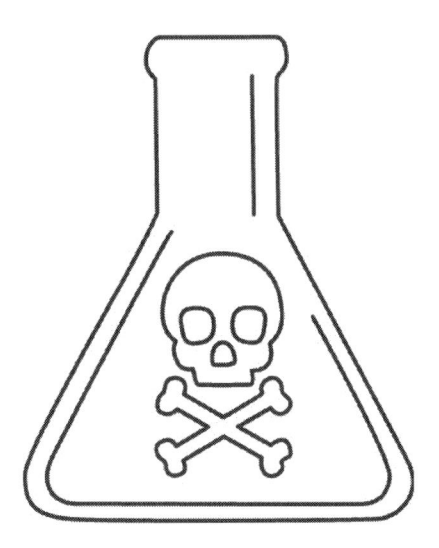

By the summer of 2015, I had already spent six long years trying to find safe and delicious gluten-free food to eat and safe products to use. I got a little help from an app called "Think Dirty." Prior to that, Lannie and I had spent countless hours understanding the chemical garble that manufacturers of clothing, makeup, shampoo, skin care, sunscreen, perfume, deodorant, and household cleaners put in their products. We had gone through so many products, I thought for sure we were finally done and had found safe options.

This new (at the time) app called Think Dirty (www.ThinkDirtyApp.com) would change everything we thought we knew about chemically free products. Now remember, we had called all the companies whose products we were using, so we felt confident.

Lannie told to me to gather up all of my makeup and expensive "safe" soaps, creams, etc., including the baby goat soap I used and my grandson used. I had bought it because it claimed to be safe for babies and my grandson had been using it for years, since he was a baby. How bad could it be? When we scanned the product it came up a TEN (10). On this scale, a ten is <u>not</u> good. It's really bad - with the highest level of the worst chemicals. I was distraught. I had given it to my grandson with eczema thinking I was giving him something beneficial.

We began to analyze all of my so-called safe products and I was shocked and sickened. Not one single product was chemical-free. My shampoo and conditioner were 3s and 4s. If zero is the best, then my hair products were moderately toxic! I kept thinking how are these companies getting away with knowing how toxic their products are for the human body? How do they get away with charging <u>extra</u> because supposedly they are safe and healthy – when in reality they are toxic?

So we had to start over again. It was like the never-ending search for non-toxic gluten free goods. It took me awhile to calm down, but once I did, I switched into research mode again.

I stopped using mouthwash with toxic chemicals and started oil pulling once a day with organic grape seed, olive, or coconut oil. Oils take the bacteria off your teeth and out of your mouth the healthy way and leave your teeth feeling good and white without chemicals. I also started to use those same oils on my skin and my skin started to get healthy. I knew for sure that pure organic oils were not going to kill me; in fact they make everything soft and smooth.

I had to switch everything I used to chemical-free and anything that I could not define, spell, or read had to be done away with. This included all dental products that contained chemicals, so most of my dental products were out. I switched to Desert Essence for toothpaste and floss (www.DesertEssence.com) and combined them with my oil pulling. I have since found another good toothpaste, Kiss My Face, which I use as well. (www.KissMyFace.com)

As this process evolved, I considered what people would have used in ancient times before all the chemicals were introduced. What did beautiful Cleopatra really use for skin care? What did she use to clean her teeth and to clean her body? For one thing she added real milk and honey to her bath water. She used real goat's milk to clean her face (not toxic goat soap), so I decided to use real goat's milk in my bath water because it contained Caprylic Capric Triglycerides to soften and moisturize the skin, just like Cleopatra. I also started using real honey and coconut oil to soften the skin on my face, hands, and feet, and coconut oil in my hair. Everything was turning softer and silkier, and less toxic.

I found out that you could use baking soda and water to cleanse your face and body. That guarantees no chemicals, is really inexpensive, and is available everywhere. If you wash with baking soda and then use milk and honey on your face you are way ahead of the game both financially and medically. If you add in mouth washing with oils you will save your teeth and gums, and spend less money. Another win-win.

## Healthy Chemical Free Soaps and Toothpastes

**Dr. Bronner's Pure-Castile Soaps** (www.DrBronner.com) There is even a Dr. Bronner's Baby Unscented Liquid Castile Soap. I have used both the baby soap and the Almond Pure-Castile liquid soap.

**Desert Essence Natural Tea Tree Oil and Neem Toothpaste with Natural Tea Tree Ginger** (www.DesertEssence.com)

**Kiss My Face Fluoride Free Whitening Toothpaste** (www.KissMyFace.com) or (www.ThriveMarket.com) This toothpaste tastes great and includes tea tree oil, Iceland moss, olive leaf extract, xylitol, silica and peppermint.

## Face Wash

I combine oil with lime to cleanse my skin and when done I combine:
1 tablespoon of honey
1 tablespoon of baking soda
1 tablespoon of sea salt
Grind into a paste and rub into the skin
Leave it on for about 4 minutes.
Rub it off and see how that it goes…also inexpensive

## Mouth Wash

I use just plain old everyday organic oil. I like sesame oil because of the smell it gives off. You can use coconut oil, which contains Medium Chain Triglycerides (a substance that will lower triglyceride cholesterol levels and raise HDL good cholesterol).

I cook with it as well. Coconut oil also contains Lauric acid, which kills all harmful pathogens, fungi, and viruses. This acid found in coconut oil can fight acne, so why not use it on the skin? Now that I know what coconut oil has done for me, I consider it a medical product for many ailments including healing your gut from e-coli.

## Frankincense Oil

Want to slow down getting wrinkles? Who doesn't? I looked into getting some work done and everything I looked into came with pretty bad side effects, so I decided to age gracefully, once I knew I was going to live!

I now mix seven drops of Frankincense oil to one ounce of my favorite pure oil and put it in a small jar. I then rub a small amount on my face daily. I put it under my eyes and around anything hanging on my face. I know this is helping me because I looked really bad after years of waiting to die in a bed. I was also told to purchase pure essential oils but I still use organic coconut oils. I love the smell of coconut, so that is what I used to mix it with. This did help with my skin and with some mild wrinkles and scarring.

*The benefits of Frankincense Oil…*
Reduce acne
Tighten skin and get rid of some wrinkles
Anxiety
Reduce stress (an epidemic in America)
Reduce inflammation
Lessen pain when rubbed on painful area
Detox

Homemade Non-Toxic Eyeliner

I found this recipe on the internet and I absolutely love it.

*Ingredients*:
Activated Charcoal Capsules (available in drugstores)
Coconut Oil (or any oil of your choice – organic of course)
Open up 1-3 charcoal capsules and pour the powder into a tiny bowl or empty eye shadow pot.
Add in a 1/2 teaspoon of coconut oil (more or less depending on how thick you want your liner to be)
Stir the charcoal and the coconut oil with your finger, a spoon, sticks or an eyeliner brush until the eyeliner is liquid and paint-like.
Store the mixture in an empty eye shadow pan or pot or any type of jar with a lid.
Use an eyeliner brush to apply the liner to your eyes and you're good to go!

There are new companies offering nontoxic products all the time, thankfully. One company came into existence because a dermatologist's wife came down with an eye disease caused by chemicals in her mascara. She was only 22 years old. Not wearing mascara bothered her so she and her husband produced their own safe mascara and started Red Apple Lipstick (www.RedAppleLipstick.com). This wonderful company carries all kinds of great makeup.

Hair Color

I use only one product and it is called Herbatint (https://usa.herbatint.com/en).

This company has been around since 1970 and their products are produced in France, where bad chemicals are banned from use. I called Herbatint and asked about lead and other chemicals that might be used in hair color, but their company actually says on the box "no ammonia, alcohol, and parabens, and safe for sensitive skin."

You can also buy Surya Brasil's Henna (www.SuryaBrasilProducts.com).These products are free of: ammonia, PPD, peroxide, parabens, resorcinol, heavy metals, mineral oil or GMOs, artificial fragrance, and gluten.

Perfume

Toxic ingredients are permitted in our products in America, but have been banned in Europe. Why is that? These are ingredients you don't want in any of the products you use, but are common in soaps, mouthwashes, makeup, nail care, and other everyday toiletries. For example, below is a list of common perfume ingredients:

Acetone
Ethanol
Benzaldehyde
Formaldehyde
Limonene
Methylene chloride
Camphor
Ethyl Acetate
Linalool
Benzyl Alcohol
Phthalates
Synthetic Musks

One time I remember distinctly two ladies joined me on an elevator and they smelled awful. They were doused in toxic perfume. I thought to myself, "come on ladies, you stink, and it's not from not showering!" Less is more and instead of spraying poison all over yourself - why not just shower? For people like me who have serious health problems, including trouble breathing, please wear perfume lightly (if you must) and understand that you are spraying pure toxic chemicals all over yourself and your loved ones. Perfumes do make people like me sick and I am not alone.

To this day, every time someone with heavy perfume comes into my elevator, I choose to get out instead of covering my face and risk being insulting. I'm not blaming them, I was the Shalimar girl in high school and I love it to this day, but I choose my health. I will wear Shalimar once in a blue moon, but only rarely. I'll settle for regular showers, coconut oil, and vanilla oil.

Deodorant

What could they possibly put in deodorant that would kill me? Well, it turns out, like everything else, plenty. My deodorant had to go because it had aluminum and other bad things in it. In its place I use gluten-free savonnerie powdered deodorant (https://gfsoap.com/GF/ProductID/32) and Crystal Deodorant (www.TheCrystal.com) which has been around for a long time.

Interestingly, since I went gluten free, took away all the foods I was intolerant too, and then detoxed my metals; I don't really need deodorant any more. I kind of smell like a clean baby because I use Dr. Bonner's soap and all the other natural products I've discovered.

Clothing

One day I was shopping at Macy's with my sister and we were trying on clothing from China. That's when the wheezing began. I was trying to figure out if I had forgotten to take all my crazy breathing medication. This was a time when I couldn't go into many stores because of the way they smelled. What I didn't know then was that the clothing in the stores was full of toxic chemicals. Clothing companies don't want their clothing looking wrinkled so they add chemicals like formaldehyde, and for people like me and Lannie, it was noticeable to the point of not being able to breathe. Many people have asthma today and they don't know what triggers it. I wanted to know why trying on clothes caused such a severe reaction in me, to the point where I couldn't consider trying them on in the store without first using my inhaler.

I used to think how crazy I had become but it was a matter of life and death for both Lannie and myself. If I was chemically sensitive, I had become that way from too many chemicals in my daily life. I didn't need big clothing stores or malls to add to my troubles. Luckily for me my body lets me know when it is too much but not everyone gets a sign.

On my search to find out what else was part of the fabric (I'm good with the puns, right?) of my clothing, I found a lot of unsavory toxins. These chemicals cause major harm to children and adults. They cause serious hormonal changes and can cause breast cancer in both women and men. I thought that just washing my clothes, (I wash everything before putting it on, including underwear), would make it better. Then I learned that washing the clothes does absolutely nothing to get rid of many toxins. The alternative was walking around in my birthday suit – not a pretty sight at my age. Many dyes cannot be washed out of the clothes and are readily absorbed into the skin. Long-term exposure does cause cancer, so in order for me to stay healthy, I had to find clothing made without dyes. Good luck right? Looks like naked it is.

Here are some of the chemicals in your clothes:

**Toxic dyes** - often called dyes. They are carcinogenic and can alter our genes!

**Formaldehyde** – used to keep clothes looking unwrinkled. Exposure to this chemical causes irritation to the throat, eyes, and lungs and can trigger asthma. This stuff can damage eyes and skin permanently.

**NPEs** - inexpensive nonionic surfactants frequently used in the global textile industry. According to Dr. Mercola (www.Mercola.com), "NPEs have, in fact, been banned already in Europe, and restricted in the United States and Canada. Even WalMart has listed NPEs as one of three chemicals they're asking suppliers to phase out. However, people will remain at risk until the chemicals are banned from the textile industry entirely. Until this time, virtually any time new clothing is washed, NPEs will be released into the environment, even in areas that have banned their use in manufacturing."

**Decomposable Aromatic Amine** - also known as azo dyes. Azo dyes are one of the main types of dye used by the textile industry. However, some azo dyes break down during use and release chemicals known as aromatic amines, some of which can cause can cancer.

**Chromium VI** - used on leather and wool and causes contact dermatitis.

**DMF** - prevents mold and moisture from building up on leather, and will exacerbate eczema.

**Dispersion Dyes** - used to make pretty colors on clothes and will cause allergies and rashes.

**Alkylphenols** - used for leather - disrupts the human endocrine system and is very toxic.

**Phthalates** - they use this to make shoes. It can disrupt the hormones in our bodies.

So once I read all this, I wondered what the hell I was going to do. How do I remove these chemicals when they were in all my clothes? I also had to stop wearing any leather products. I kept learning and here is what I have to do. I no longer shop in stores that reek of those funky smells that make my breathing go haywire. I can smell a bad store a few feet from the entrance – so I don't even go in.

**When I buy new clothes I always:**
Wash everything *three* times before I wear it.

I never go to the dry cleaners. I buy only washable clothing.

I don't buy products that are water or stain resistant unless I write to the company to find out exactly what they use in processing their stuff.

I shop for natural textiles like cotton and linen. I even have cotton and chemical-free sheets.

I just know that if we become educated and stop buying low quality stuff from China, our bodies and minds will be healthier. California and India make cotton clothing, 100% chemical free. This may be more expensive, but one option is to buy less of everything and take better care of it. Also, the alternative to chemical-free clothing and bedding is illness, which as we all know is extremely expensive in the U.S. It is work to find the stuff, and it is pricier, but the end result is well worth it. For me, I am here among the living, thriving, dancing, and not hooked up to breathing machines every day, unable to leave my home.

Further Reading

If you are reading the paperback instead of the ebook - you can type each title below in your computer search bar and find the referenced article.

Should You Try Oil Pulling?

The Ultimate Guide To Clean Beauty

15 Toxic Ingredients To Avoid In Skincare Products

The Hidden Dangers Of Makeup And Shampoo

7 Harmful Ingredients In Your Deodorant

Is Modern Life Poisoning Me?

Customers Beware: Toxins Lurking In Your Clothing!

# 20

# CHOCOLATE EXPOSED

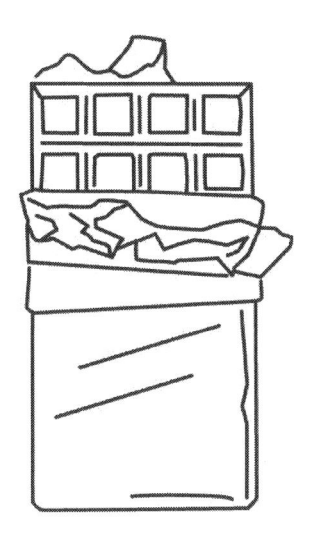

Chocolate is such a beloved food in America. It's tasty and seems to have some medicinal properties. As I searched for things that wouldn't make me sick, chocolate seemed like a good place to start. I needed it to be gluten free and that took some doing, but after a week I was able to find something I deemed acceptable. I began to eat Dove and Musketeers. (I needed something that would raise my blood sugar in case it went really low and this is why I chose candy). These are both gluten free and I found that chocolate decreased stroke risk, improved blood flow, and might prevent blood clots - so far, so good. It also works on the brain cells and makes them healthier, and everyone needs more brain cells, especially at my age. If chocolate helped I was in!

Of course, you have to wonder who is doing this research and coming up with these findings – chocolate manufacturers perhaps? I also read that people who ate chocolate had prettier skin, so I was into this as my wrinkles were starting to show and we all know how much women hate wrinkles. Chocolate also has plenty of antioxidants, flavonoids, and polyphenols that promote anti-aging. Aging in America is a crime, so anything to prevent it. Chocolate can make us more relaxed because it has been know to increase our brain waves and it does raise our serotonin levels. At first glance, chocolate has a lot going for it. It was not on my "to eat" list. In fact, it was something I hadn't eaten in 34 years as a type 1 diabetic. But things changed once I went gluten free. The major blood sugar swings weren't as bad now and my body could handle a piece of chocolate.

I purchased a new drink made from cocoa but cooked up like coffee called Crio Bru. I loved this stuff and I got a break from drinking coffee every day. I continued to rotate foods to avoid food intolerances. This cocoa drink seemed like a good addition to the rotation. I had coffee one day, cocoa the next, and then tea.

Things were going great until late one night I heard someone on TV talking about the dangers of eating chocolate. I said out loud to no one in particular, "really and now this too?" What in the world could possibly be in my wonderful chocolate drink that is going to kill me…except maybe the soy that is in every single chocolate product? Sadly my morning cocoa was about to change and my warning light went on. Chocolate might be harmful to my body too. I was too exhausted to think about it that night but I knew the following morning was going to be disappointing. Would there be anything safe left for unsuspecting people to eat or drink?

The next morning I began my search for the evils of chocolate. After one hour I sat on my couch shocked. My journey to understand what I was both eating and drinking disturbed me and I ended up sad and frustrated. I was paying a good deal of money to drink cadmium, arsenic, and lead for my morning breakfast. You know what makes me angry? The FDA knows full well what we are ingesting and they encourage it because it is profitable for the company selling the product. They make excuses and say something stupid about chocolate having allowable levels of those heavy metals. This is all about money and since the FDA doesn't regulate any food companies in America they can feed you as many heavy metals as possible…and they are.

The first article I read was about Hershey's, Mars, and See's candies containing heavy metals, but at low doses. It also said that the levels were too low to cause any harm. So here I was having a breakfast drink with low levels of three very toxic ingredients. I threw my hands up in disgust and waited until 10:00 a.m. to call Crio Bru to see if they were testing for heavy metals. I spoke with a company representative and she assured me that they checked their products for toxic ingredients like cadmium and lead, and last year's tests came out clean. I sighed with relief and then asked for a copy of the test results. She agreed to send them to me, but six months later I was still waiting. I never got those results so I gave up that drink.

Next I called my favorite chocolate company, Enjoy Life, and they talked me through their research on heavy metals. I love that company and continue to make delicious candies out of their chocolate (www.EnjoyLifeFoods.com). I recommend Enjoy Life Chocolate, only dark.

Want something easy to make from Enjoy Life's Dare Chocolate?

### *Gail's Recipe for a Candy Bar.*
Melt the Enjoy Life chocolate, and add nuts, cranberries, coconut, orange peel, rice cereal, or any thing else you think you might want to put into it.

Pour it onto parchment paper and put into the refrigerator to harden. Wait at least 2 hours then break it up into pieces.

Store that in a glass container and keep in the refrigerator for at least two months if it lasts that long without being devoured!

You now have healthy candy bars without any heavy metals…except maybe the rice cereal. My life has become one big science and research experiment and the irony is my worst subject in school was science.

I can no longer just buy something without doing research. Everything I purchase is always preceded by a phone call to the company. This can be a pain in the butt, especially in the midst of a very busy life, but it is worth it because of how I feel and look today. I know 70 isn't 48, but I look and act younger than many of my friends, and some of them are ten years younger than me! I know that what I have done made me well and keeps me well.

As it turns out, some huge chocolate producers were hit with a lawsuit in 2014 accusing them of violating California's Safe Drinking Water & Toxic Enforcement Act of 1986 by exposing their consumers to lead and cadmium, known toxic chemicals. Some of the companies sued were Ghirardelli, Hershey, Godiva, Lindt, Green & Black's, and Earth Circle Organics. That lawsuit was settled finally in 2018 forcing chocolate manufacturers to determine what was causing these contaminations and take steps to reduce these toxic ingredients in their chocolate products. I don't know about you, but reduce isn't good enough for me. I don't want any toxic chemicals in my chocolate, which is why I choose Enjoy Life.

Further Reading

If you are reading the paperback instead of the ebook - you can type each title below in your computer search bar and find the referenced article.

Toxic Chocolate

Court Establishes Guidelines For Chocolate Sold In California

Killing At Source: How To Avoid Cadmium And Lead In Chocolate

## 21

## CORN – THE GMO KIND

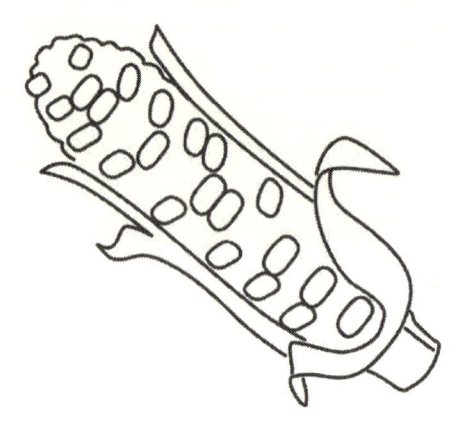

During one of my research episodes, I decided to look up some articles on certain organic foods. I was disappointed. I pay a good deal of money to be safe from the poisons that big companies want to put into my body, and here was another curve ball. Every time I let my guard down, I discover I can't. But I can't do it alone. We all need to stand up to the American way of producing our processed foods. If we don't then I'm sorry to say we deserve what they are dishing out.

In the San Diego Free Press I came upon an article written by John Lawrence of Social Choice and Beyond. The title of the article was "Who Knew? Organic Foods Contain a Dose of GMO's." Really America? For people like me who cannot tolerate GMOs, I find this particularly disturbing and the fact that they keep it a secret is downright scary. In the article he writes, "to be labeled as 'USDA Organic,' 95% of the ingredients must be organically grown and the remaining 5% may be non-organic agricultural ingredients or synthetic substances that have been approved for use in organics by the USDA."

I continue to read that America has allowed 5% to be a GMO made from corn. This is the one food that I have been trying to get out of my system. I do not want corn in my digestive track to screw up what I have been trying to fix for so many years. To add insult to injury, I had started to call companies that listed an ingredient called "organic citric acid" because I had gotten sick from a vitamin pill that contained it. I came to find out that citric acid is not made from fruit. It is made from a very bad cheap corn. Now when I see it on an organic ingredient list, like the applesauce I just returned, I call the company and ask what it is derived from. When I hear silence and they say they will call me back, I thank them, hang up, and return the product. Poison in our foods has many names. This kind of citric acid will cause digestive problems and erode the enamel off your teeth.

Corn was purple once upon a time, and all foods that naturally contain the color purple are higher in flavonoids and resveratrol. If corn were still purple it would be a healthy food choice, unless of course you are me and intolerant to eating it no matter what the color. I have not eaten corn or wheat for at least 10 years because both those foods make my hair fall out. I am not saying that corn has no value because it does contain lutein and zeaxanthin and can grow good gut bacteria which helps with digestion. That being said it raises blood sugar off the charts and as corn gets whiter it gets higher in carbs. It has a higher glycemic load prompting Harvard researchers to call it the unhealthiest vegetable you can eat. The blood sugar spikes people experience after eating corn act like a drug and cause them to eat even more. This is a bad carb! The problem I had with keeping it out of my diet was the many ways companies hid this GMO product in their food.

I avoided cold cuts at the grocery store for many years due to my gluten issues. But then I learned that I could ask that the slicer be cleaned prior to slicing my meat and cheese, so I felt satisfied with that and decided to try cold cuts again. I chose Board's Head chicken, thinking it was a quality product. They cleaned the machine and sliced four pieces for me. I felt secure.

Within four hours of eating my first store-purchased cold cut from Boar's Head my hair started falling out! I didn't get the kind of sick feeling that comes from eating gluten, but I knew something had invaded my system and I had to get to the bottom of it. I was not going to risk losing my hair again under any circumstances. I was so upset and horrified to learn that Boar's Head was hiding GMO corn in their products by calling it dextrose. I got on the phone again. I gave them five minutes to tell me the truth and eventually they told me that their dextrose was corn syrup. It was appalling. Shame on Boar's Head. Another disappointment and another lesson learned.

I always encourage everyone to read labels of course, but now you need to keep a list of ingredients companies are trying to hide by calling them something else. Be aware if you have autoimmune diseases, corn should be off the menu. And let's be real, if corn was not so bad why do the big companies hide their use of it? Why didn't Boar's Head call their dextrose "corn syrup" or just "corn dextrose?" Why doesn't the Food and Drug

Administration (FDA) put corn down as an allergen like they do wheat? If that were the case then companies would have to admit to their use of it no matter how it was worded. I don't know why corn has to be in so many products, but it should be labeled so people like me don't get sick when eating something they think is safe. If it's labeled, the individual consumer can make an educated decision whether to eat it or not.

A final thought, when a label says "natural," that means absolutely nothing. There is nothing natural about natural foods in this country.

Further Reading

If you are reading the paperback instead of the ebook - you can type each title below in your computer search bar and find the referenced article.

This Is The Unhealthiest Vegetable You Can Eat, According To Harvard Scientists

What You Need To Know About GMOs

Hidden Corn Based Ingredients

Leader Of Largest US Organic Food Fraud Gets 10-Year Term

## 22

## FISH – SOMETHING'S FISHY

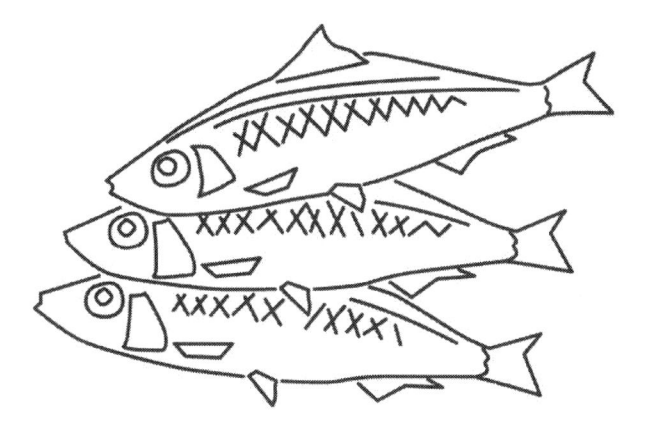

What can you do to ensure that the fish you buy and eat is safe and providing enough Omega 3s (about 500 mg/day) without ingesting more toxins? The first step is to know where your fish comes from. You won't be able to count on the government to protect you. Greed will keep toxic fish in the marketplace. You'll have to get educated to stay healthy.

It's a fact that our waters are polluted and we have been advised against eating certain fish too often. Most farm-raised seafood is <u>not</u> a healthy choice and yet because of water pollution, some farm-raised products are now better for us than wild. For example, I no longer want any shrimp from the Gulf of Mexico or from the west coast of Florida. They used to be my first choice. Every time I want to eat fish I look up which are the least toxic fish, where they are from, and if they are farm-raised.

The levels of mercury in our ocean fish will most definitely go up in the next ten years and it is coming out of Asia. The type of mercury poisoning our system is called methylmercury and it is the most toxic. I now only buy my fish from certain parts of Alaska and Washington and only from companies that are testing their products. So now the question is which fish should I eat and how often?

It seems that big predatory fish go deeper into the ocean and eat the most toxins. Too much exposure to methylmercury will adversely affect the human body. The goal is to avoid that at all costs.

Here is a partial fish list:
**Do not eat**: swordfish
**Eat Sometimes**: tuna
**Eat frequently but only wild**: salmon, cod, sole, clams
**Eat often**: Sardines, farm raised shrimp from America, and none from other countries

## Further Reading

If you are reading the paperback instead of the ebook - you can type each title below in your computer search bar and find the referenced article.

Scientists Pinpoint Source Of Mercury In Pacific Ocean Fish

Study Tracks Mercury Sources In Seafood

Health Effects Of Exposures To Mercury

# 23

# GLUTEN ALMOST KILLED ME – WHAT COULD IT BE DOING TO YOU?

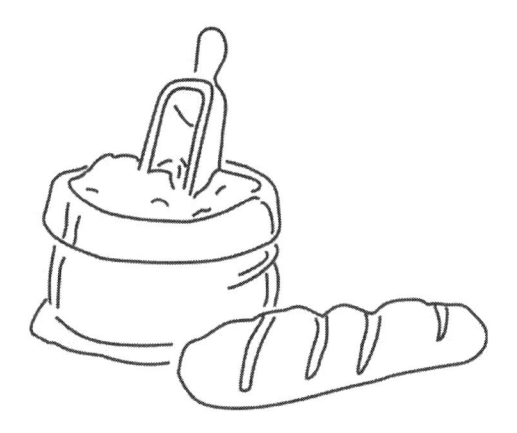

More than a decade ago, it would have been hard for me to wrap my head around the fact that my vegetarian diet filled with supposedly healthy grains and a lot of whole wheat, some fish, eggs, cheese, nuts, fruits, and vegetables, was not so healthy. For a type 1 diabetic, I was convinced it was a great diet, closely resembling the storied Mediterranean diet, olive oil and all. When I started having severe allergies and the autoimmune problems exploded, I never thought it could be related to the food choices I was making.

No one spoke of gluten and its connection to autoimmune diseases ten years ago. No one spoke of gluten at all. The only way I could figure out what to do with my eating was the research coming out of Europe and Canada. In America, doctors only treat symptoms and diseases with prescriptions. The concept of healing through healthy food choices is seemingly beyond the comprehension of the medical community. They refuse to look at the causes of disease.

When alopecia came into my life, something in me just clicked. I was undergoing cortisone shots in my head every week for a year, and still losing the battle. At the time, I didn't know that cortisone could cause cataracts because no one mentioned the possible trade-offs with that treatment. At the end of the day, the big reveal was that no one could help me. I had to help myself. I was determined to understand the <u>why</u> of what was happening and not obsess about this and that treatment. My body was inflamed and I needed to somehow put out the fire.

Who could imagine that my research and testing, on both Lannie and myself, was going to find the answer – gluten. Gluten was one of the causes of my alopecia and all the other autoimmune problems I had. I was desperate to keep my hair and I didn't want any more autoimmune diseases to join the party. I wrote this book, not to preach, but to present an alternative. I cannot tell anyone what to do, nor do I want to, but I can tell you what I now know to be true. Lannie, Larry, and I decided to give it a shot and the results speak for themselves. It wasn't an easy or hassle-free road, but it was certainly worthwhile.

I went gluten free for the first three plus years and when I didn't see the results I wanted, I went grain free. I am not a doctor but I do know that once I went grain free my body started the healing process. It took Lannie and I years to heal. Total healing doesn't happen overnight. It takes patience and persistence. Humans destroy their gut microbes by eating mega-doses of sugar, dead dairy made from very sickly cows (there is nothing healthy in the cow's milk from America which contains blood and pus), and then all the other processed foods that include toxic chemicals.

I began to include in my diet probiotics from fermented vegetables that I make at home, powdered collagen peptides from Vital Proteins ([www.VitalProteins.com](www.VitalProteins.com)), organic bone broth, Camu Powder from Navitas ([www.NavitasOrganics.com](www.NavitasOrganics.com)), and Glutamine. I roasted my own grass-fed beef, sliced it, and froze it into serving sizes. I was able to buy a great deal of fresh turkey without the added gluten, corn, sugar, and soy for a lot less money than $10/lb. We as Americans are too lazy to throw a piece of turkey in a crockpot, cover it, and wait for eight hours for the final product. We choose to eat processed cold cuts and other garbage instead. Sorry Boar's Head, you put GMO corn in your products under the false name of dextrose, but don't tell anyone it is corn. You only fess up when you get a nasty phone call from Gluten Free Gail!

Now, in 2019, more and more people are turning to a gluten-free diet for many health reasons. News about grains being a poison to the body is coming out every day, but not enough information is hitting the doctors' offices - where it needs to be. It seems they didn't get the memo about the dangers of SAD (standard American diet), and facts about how to eat healthy grains is not in the books yet.

When I speak of why grains are causing inflammation, very few people take it seriously. People cannot imagine that the healthy wheat the FDA pushed on us beginning in early childhood is actually making us <u>sick</u> and not keeping us <u>well</u>. Please understand that wheat is not the only factor involved in making Americans fatter and sicker, but it does play a role in the health of all Americans. Some people are unable to digest this type of product due to an unhealthy gut flora and the change in wheat's chromosomes over the last several decades.

For me to get healthy I had to address each issue, one at a time. Here are the facts about the wheat eaten and other grains like rye and barley. Each grain has a different gluten structure of proteins. One is called Gliadin and the other is called Glutenin. All grains contain prolamins - which is why when people just stop eating *wheat* they do not get well right away.

What is a Prolamin? Here is the Wikipedia definition.

**Prolamins** are a group of plant <u>storage proteins</u> having a high <u>proline</u> content and found in the seeds of cereal grains: <u>wheat</u> (<u>gliadin</u>), <u>barley</u> (<u>hordein</u>), <u>rye</u> (<u>secalin</u>), <u>corn</u> (<u>zein</u>), <u>sorghum</u> (<u>kafirin</u>) and as a minor protein, <u>avenin</u> in <u>oats</u>. They are characterized by a high <u>glutamine</u> and <u>proline</u> content and are generally soluble only in strong <u>alcohol</u> solutions. Some prolamins, notably <u>gliadin</u>, and similar proteins found in the tribe Triticeae (see <u>Triticeae glutens</u>) may induce <u>celiac disease</u> in genetically predisposed individuals.

| GRAINS | PROLAMINS |
|---|---|
| Wheat | Gliadin |
| Rye | Secalin |
| Sorghum | Kafirin |
| Oats | Avenin |
| Barley | Hordein |
| Corn | Zein |

Here is the reason I went grain free for years. I knew that if I wasn't responding enough to the gluten-free diet that I had another choice and I was going to do whatever it took. During those years I was able to make bread from green pea flour, banana flour, almond flour, coconut flour, plantains, chickpea flour and one of my favorites, buckwheat flour. I made bread, which I fermented using buckwheat so it would rise without man-made yeasts, and it was delicious. I made sweet potato rolls and they too were wonderful. I managed to live without the grains for three years. I didn't miss them or skip a beat as I made rolls, muffins, flatbreads and crackers with my grain-free flours. Some of these flours are very high in both protein and fiber. Coffee flour, pea, coconut, chickpea, buckwheat, and plantains are higher in fiber than the normal everyday wheat products and much more digestible.

The changing of the wheat chromosomes is one of the factors in gluten intolerance and the rise in celiac disease. Wheat went from two chromosomes to eight, too many for a lot of us. When those wheat prolamins hit the gut they leach into our blood stream and cause autoimmune diseases. The other factor is Round-Up and Glyphosates that are sprayed on all our grains and manufactured by Monsanto. Monsanto owns the FDA, EPA, and now WEBMD, which makes me very sad. The chemical Glyphosate was brought on the market in 1976 to kill weeds but instead it is killing us. Our bodies cannot remove all those chemicals when we eat them every day.

There are more discussions today about wheat and celiac disease, but what about those people who have severe gluten intolerance and cannot be diagnosed? Finally, some research has come down the pike about something called "non-celiac gluten sensitivity." Celiac disease is not a food allergy. It's an autoimmune disease. And although Lannie and I have plenty of autoimmune diseases, celiac is probably not one of them. But we definitely have a severe gluten sensitivity. However, at this point gluten is so dangerous, no one should eat it.

I am happy to say there are no prescription drugs required to treat celiac disease or gluten sensitivity. The only protocol is to stay away from gluten. There are 300 symptoms of gluten intolerance and if you have too many symptoms just go gluten free. Gluten affects every single organ in the body including the blood, and avoiding it is the best medicine.

Further Reading

If you are reading the paperback instead of the ebook - you can type each title below in your computer search bar and find the referenced article.

Could Gluten Be Causing Your Health Problems?

The Connection Between Gluten And Neuropathy

Why A Low-Gluten Diet May Benefit Everyone

## 24

## GLYPHOSATE – BE AFRAID, BE VERY AFRAID

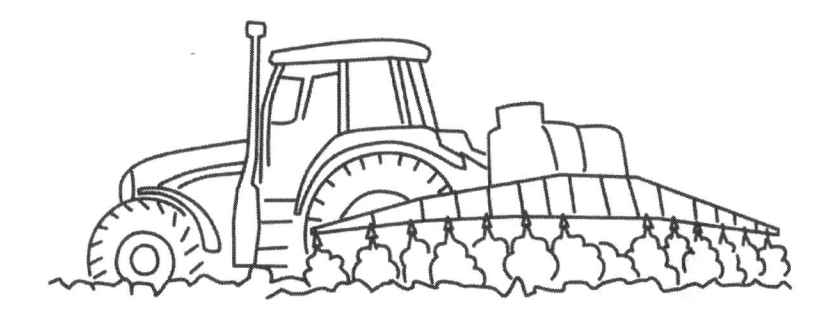

It is important that we as Americans have factual information from reliable sources. I was using WebMD because I felt that they had nothing to do with big business and then this showed up on my computer from Dr. Mercola who I absolutely trust. The headline was: "WebMD Implicated in Cancer Coverup." I sat up and shook my head hoping I could clear the fog I was in. WebMD was my go-to site and now this?

I also found out that Monsanto was paying off the Director of Nutrition for WebMD. This was so disturbing. Her job was to discuss how wonderful Monsanto's products were, which we all know they are not, and she did it. Is there no one we can trust to give us real factual information so we can be better educated and make healthy choices for our families? For me it means I must find another source of health information to pass on to people.

Monsanto is really dangerous. Could the news get any worse about Glyphosate, otherwise known as Round-Up? They spray it on our farmland and make every single thing in our environment toxic.

As of April 2017 there were 150 new lawsuit cases filed against Monsanto and in California, the use of Glyphosate on farmland has been labeled a carcinogen – known to cause cancer. That being said, the EPA is still permitting the use of this cancer-causing agent on all our grains. This is why when people ask me how I can do without my daily dose of bread and pasta I laugh. I know what is being used to grow it faster and without sprouting. Do I miss what America is eating? Not a chance.

So now the EPA, FDA, and WebMD are all on the take? Who is left? I use Dr. Mercola for a good deal of real information (www.DrMercola.com). I use my fish company Vital Choice (www.VitalChoice.com) for factual information about many topics. I also go to Dr. Ron's (www.DrRons.com) who sells healthy vitamins and writes about many things that pertain to our health. The information is out there. We just have to know who is telling the truth and who hasn't sold out.

Further Reading

If you are reading the paperback instead of the ebook - you can type each title below in your computer search bar and find the referenced article.

The Weed Killer In Our Food Is Killing Us

EPA Official Accused Of Helping Monsanto Kill Cancer Study

Bayer Granted Request To Move Some Glyphosate Trials Out Of California

New Home Test Kit Enables Easy Glyphosate Detection

# 25

# HEAVY METAL – NOT THE MUSIC, THE POISON

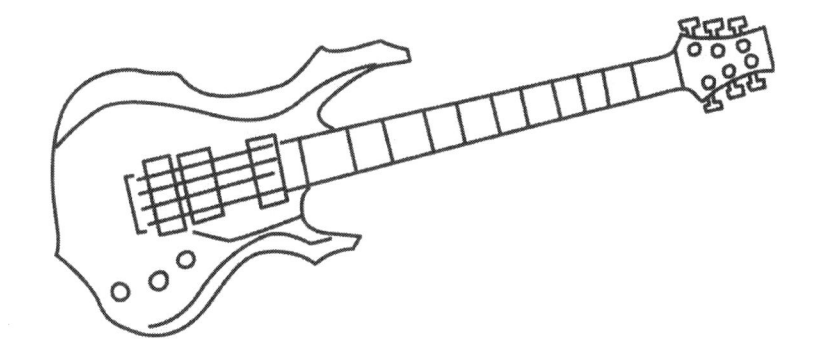

Even today, in 2019, I am still wondering how any of us manage to stay healthy with all the bad stuff in our environment. When I went gluten free in 2009, I thought my story was over. I was healing and getting better all the time. But in 2016 I faced another health crisis. I came down with a sickly gallbladder and chemical toxins showed up in my urine.

How did someone like me who carefully read every item on the ingredient list show up with heavy metals in both her urine and blood? I am calmer today about both things but included this in my guide so anyone reading it can get all the facts. I was not calm when I first got the test results!

The initial question I asked myself was where would I get both arsenic and cadmium in my blood and urine? I went back to the drawing board and thought about what I had done differently. I went through my kitchen and came back with the new organic brown rice I was using to make sourdough starter and sourdough gluten-free breads. I glanced over at the flax meal I was about to make into crackers. These were the only new things I had been eating. I called Arrowhead Mills and asked about their levels of arsenic and they advised me to look online. I knew that was a bad sign because if everything was ok, they would have told me. After hours spent researching, I found my culprit. It was Arrowhead Mills Organic Brown Rice. This product had(s) one the highest levels of arsenic, so one down and one to go.

My next challenge was to find out why flax caused me to have cadmium in my blood stream. To my dismay, I found out that California and parts of Canada have the highest levels of cadmium in both their air and the ground. Most flax comes from both California and Canada. This is what I had added to my diet to increase my Omega 3s!

I wanted to go further and find out what heavy metals did to the body. I knew they produced cataracts, but what other kinds of damage did they do and how fast could I get them out? Fear was taking over and I knew that fear was not my answer, education was. So I kept studying.

The first article I read made me happy that we didn't eat food that contained fructose in my house. High fructose corn syrup is found in almost all processed food and corn is something I have not eaten in years. Sometimes I am so glad I had to give up gluten because once I did that, I had to give up processed food. At the end of this chapter I list some of the articles that I read to understand everything I could about heavy metals and where they can be found.

Cadmium and lead can be found in many chocolate products. To me this is so sad because children eat it all the time. Contamination can begin at the growing point, processing point, or during fermenting. Oftentimes it happens during manufacturing. I ate a lot of cocoa products because I thought they were a safe food and high in antioxidants. Boy was I wrong (see Chocolate chapter).

A good deal of the land used to grow products in California is loaded with cadmium. I was using flax flour from California when I learned this. Flax oil, flour, pasta, crackers, or anything made from flax is going to be highly contaminated with cadmium. This was going to be hard, but I wanted this poison out of my system and I was determined. I began by eating broken cell wall chlorella tablets that I got from Sunfood Superfoods (www.SunFood.com). These tablets are made to detox and alkalize the human body. I added organic parsley and cilantro and started using an infrared sauna and three months later both my blood and urine tests had returned to normal without Chelation Therapy. I sat down and cried with relief.

Now I eat all the things that detox the human body. We as consumers cannot get away from what is being done to our world or our products, but we can get educated and stop eating what is poisoning us. I know that organic is the only way to lessen pesticides, but I also know that the human body does not need to use plastic bottles or tin foil. Both of these things add toxins to our bodies. The goal is detoxification and it's ongoing. I use ZRT Labs to test my urine and Quest Diagnostics to test my blood.

### Foods That Detox the Human Body Naturally

Black sesame seeds only

Broken cell wall Chlorella Tablets
Fresh Organic parsley
Fresh Organic Cilantro
Cloves

Cadmium and Lead Exposure

The main route of human lead and cadmium exposure occurs via food ingestion as well as contaminated water and soil. Lead and cadmium in food are ubiquitous and do not seem to discriminate between natural, certified organic, and non-organic products. One or both of these metals has been found in various foods including baby foods (made with carrots, peaches, pears, sweet potatoes), dietary supplements, vitamins, protein powders, seaweed snacks, ginger cookies, packaged peaches/pears, various fruit juices, as well as chocolate.

Another way we are exposed to lead and cadmium is through inhalation from dust or pollution from industrial processes. Additionally, cadmium is present in cigarette smoke. The struggle is real and ongoing.

Further Reading

If you are reading the paperback instead of the ebook - you can type each title below in your computer search bar and find the referenced article.

Do You Need A Heavy Metal Detox?

Yes, There Is Arsenic In Your Rice. Here's What You Need To Know.

Cadmium Pigments In Consumer Products And Their Health Risks

## 26

# IT AIN'T HONEY, HONEY

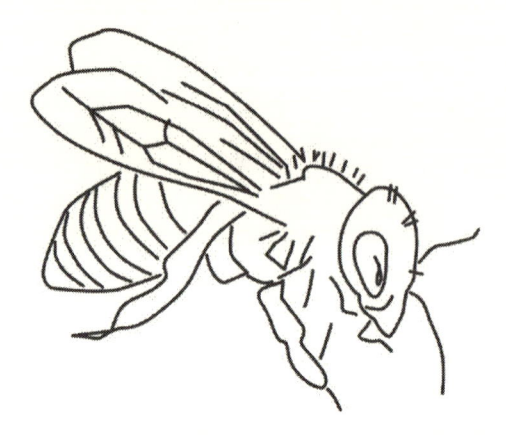

The day I found out about honey started out just like any other day. I was getting ready to ferment buckwheat grouts and decided to make a different kind of fermented bread that required honey. That is when my entire process went to hell. I just wanted a good healthy honey to add to my new bread recipe and that is why I started researching honey. Who knew honey wasn't always the real deal? Nothing for me is ever easy, but once I get to the bottom of my quest and find the safe options, I am good to go.

So, why am I talking about honey? It just comes from bees, right? That's what I thought until I started my research. I learned that honey was banned in Europe because it was toxic, yet it's still being sold in America. Sounds familiar. We permit our people to use honey that is tainted with illegal antibiotics and heavy metals.

It's all about money. Established honey packers want to save a penny and keep that money. It is now called honey smuggling and these bad people have even gone so far as to make honey that isn't even made by bees. In 2003 Chinese honey was tested in America and was found to have many contaminants, one of which can cause leukemia.

Once the powers that be did become aware of bad toxins in Chinese honey, we stopped purchasing it. But it took company recalls and people getting sick. The Chinese are smart and all they did once we stopped purchasing their honey was sell it to India where they mixed it with other stuff and sold it right back to America!

We also came up with a way to extend the shelf life of honey by filtering it and leaving it void of any nutrients or bee pollen. So don't buy this garbage unless you are looking for an unhealthy dose of fructose.

I began a search for real honey without chemicals and plastic. The fake honey had to go. And it should leave your diet as well. It can cause diabetes and obesity because of all the fructose in it. This fructose is made from that dastardly GMO corn, my arch nemesis. It may also contain antibiotics and who needs that on a daily basis? Fructose leads to plaque in the blood vessels; this alone causes heart disease.

I searched for a local honey maker that jarred their honey and didn't put it in toxic plastic containers. I discovered my best bet was organic raw honey if it could be found locally. I also learned about a product called Manuka honey, which came from Australia, and I knew that Australia made some of the healthiest and safest products. You can buy it from various online retailers.

My first purchase was the Organic Manuka honey made in a glass jar. That set me back $45.00 for 11.5 oz. Health is expensive, but disease is more expensive. They also have honey in plastic containers, which I don't understand. I say shame on them. I also purchased Tupelo Honey, which you can get on Amazon and Cloister Whipped Honey with Cinnamon from (www.CloisterHoney.com).

The benefits of raw organic honey are many. Honey is packed with vitamins, enzymes, and nutrients, it helps with allergies and for me, it stabilizes my blood sugar and blood pressure. My biggest concern was my gut and real honey and <u>only</u> real honey has the enzymes necessary to heal the gut and promote a good digestive system. I'm glad I found out the truth, because I use the good stuff now almost daily in my home.

Further Reading

If you are reading the paperback instead of the ebook - you can type each title below in your computer search bar and find the referenced article.

10 Benefits Of Manuka Honey

Chinese Honey: Banned In Europe, Is Flooding US Grocery Shelves. Here's How To Know The Difference.

Honey Tests Reveal Global Contamination By Bee-Harming Pesticides

# 27

# NUTS, A NO NO

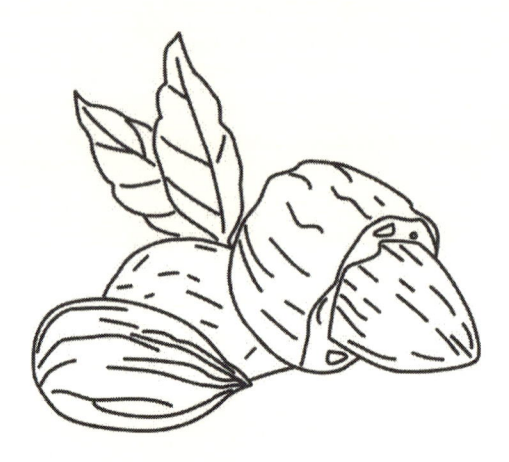

So while sitting in a timeshare I decided to order nuts on the computer. I was focused on making sure they were gluten free. Now I know that sounds weird because nuts don't contain gluten, but I would prefer to know that the nuts I buy are not sitting in a factory loaded with wheat or corn flour.

I decided to type into the search bar, "should the nuts I buy be organic too," thinking how silly that sounded. I sat and waited for my information to come up, and since this is a chapter in my book, you can imagine the results.

Nuts should, and can, be a healthy choice of proteins and vitamins, but once again America, your regular nuts are toxic and if that isn't sad enough so are all the nuts butters you purchase unless they say one word…ORGANIC.

Not all nuts contain massive amounts of toxins so let me start with the ones I know are loaded and not safe for human consumption. However, I do still believe that all nuts should be organic due to the nature of the harmful pesticides and toxins.

Cashews
Walnuts

Macadamia nuts
Pistachios
Peanuts

Almonds are a whole other story due to their treatment. Almonds are now pasteurized, and America has been doing that since 2007. There are four ways to pasteurize these beloved nuts and that is: steaming, roasting, blanching, or treating them with a very toxic fumigation treatment. Propylene oxide (PPO) is the chemical of choice. Human exposure to this chemical causes respiratory and eye irritation. If it comes in contact with the skin it causes irritation and necrosis. It can affect the nervous system and cause tumors. The EPA has labeled this chemical as a probable human carcinogen. Time to throw out all of your non-organic nuts!

I should point out here that it's perfectly legal to spray toxin-containing pesticides on almonds and for the nuts themselves to contain pesticide residues. The United States Environmental Protection Agency (EPA) sets the food standards here, and pesticides get routinely reviewed for regulatory reasons. For example, they currently allow about 20 parts per billion (20 ppb) levels of pesticide and other toxins to show up in the nuts themselves. This tolerance level would legally allow about 120 micrograms of the pesticide to show up in one cup of your almonds.

Should you risk this level of pesticide exposure by selecting non-organic almonds? The answer depends on how often you eat almonds, how many other potential toxins your body has to process, your overall level of health, and the specific health of your body's detoxification systems. In general, if you are extremely vital and healthy and don't have many other toxins for your body to process, these numbers won't bother you too much. However, if you do not have a healthy detoxification system, or you are exposed to many other routine toxins (not necessarily involving your food), a relatively small amount of pesticide residues in your almonds may increase your risk of health problems. But think of how much people actually consume when they drink almond milk or eat almond cake and ice cream. I cannot even wrap my head around this information. I know that eating organic is expensive but so are doctors and medicine. Organic is the way to go, and raw is even better.

Further Reading

If you are reading the paperback instead of the ebook - you can type each title below in your computer search bar and find the referenced article.

Is There Engine Fuel On Your Almonds?

Down To The Crunch: The Hidden Health Dangers Of Nuts

GAIL KEEHN DVORETZ

Another Reason You Shouldn't Go Nuts On Nuts

# 28

# ORGANIC ALL THE WAY

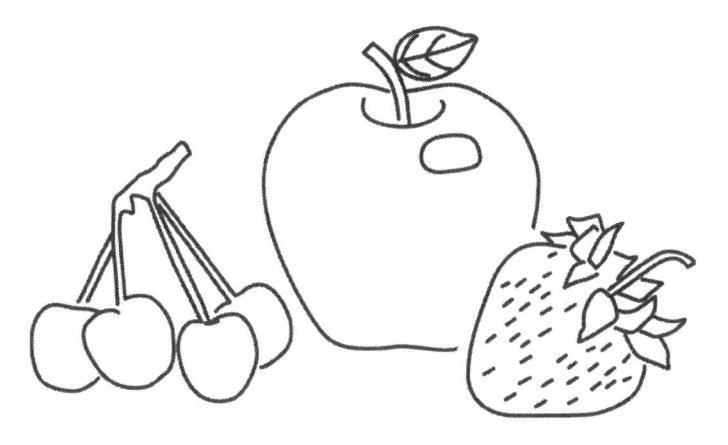

Like all humans, I never gave anything much thought until it affected me physically, mentally, or financially. Now I urge people to start <u>before</u> they get sick. Few listen, but I say it anyway. If you are reading this book, maybe you'll listen.

In order to deal with my allergies, I searched for a specialist trained in environmental allergies. It would be a miracle to find someone who knew anything about chemical intolerances and allergies. I didn't think to ask my sister, who had the same issues, and had been using a doctor near my house with those much-needed certifications. I was lucky when my sister Lannie looked up Dr. Robbins to see if he was still practicing. He was, and his office was in Deerfield Beach, FL, five miles from my house. I did my doctor-finding due diligence and he had the highest possible rating.

I knew I had found my doctor from the very first phone conversation. When the nurse called to confirm my appointment, she said, "Please don't wear perfumes, scented shampoos, soaps, or conditioners in the office. Our clients have very bad allergies." There would be no toxic chemical air fresheners in Dr. Robbins' waiting room. A miracle.

Dr. Robbins was my lifesaver because back then I was drowning in chemicals and didn't know where to begin. He knew to get me started with

Vitamin B12 shots and Vitamin D. He addressed many of my major health issues with just those two things. To this day I still give myself B12 shots, sit in the sun each day and take a Vitamin D pill. You know how I hate shots, so this is how important I believe these are. I get my levels checked all the time and so should everyone else.

Dr. Robbins suggested buying organic so I could get the pesticides out of my food, and therefore out of my bloodstream, as soon as possible. He was speaking my language. I started with the "Dirty Dozen" fruits and vegetables, which I list in this chapter. Ten years ago there were only twelve but today those chemically laden fruits and vegetables comprise a much larger list. It was an easy decision for me to make, as all healthy decisions have been when it really mattered. I was able to afford the healthy stuff because I cooked and ate almost exclusively at home.

Everyone I spoke to pointed out how much more expensive organic was. I fired back that my medical bills were taking a nosedive and I was taking less and less medication in general. At home, we adjusted our portions to reflect true serving sizes, so we were able to buy organic grass-fed protein. If one pound of beef can be made into four servings instead of two, everyone can afford better products and get thinner while doing it!

Here is the 2019 list of Dirty Dozen provided by the Environmental Working Group (www.ewg.org):

Strawberries
Spinach
Kale
Nectarines
Apples
Grapes
Peaches
Cherries
Pears
Tomatoes
Celery
Potatoes

The next list is considered "Clean Fifteen" fruits and vegetables:

Avocados
Sweet Corn
Pineapples
Frozen Sweet Peas
Onions

Papayas
Eggplant
Asparagus
Kiwis
Cabbages
Cauliflower
Cantaloupes
Broccoli
Mushrooms
Honeydew Melons

To help consumers make informed decisions, EWG updates its *Shopper's Guide to Pesticides in Produce* each year, ranking pesticide contamination on 48 popular fruits and vegetables. ([www.ewg.org](www.ewg.org)).

What more can I say about this topic except that if you want to get as many toxic pesticides out of your body and the bodies of those you love, keep an eye on these lists. Don't be fooled by how pretty those berries are. If they are not organic, they are poison.

Further Reading

If you are reading the paperback instead of the ebook - you can type each title below in your computer search bar and find the referenced article.

Even Harvard Urges Eating Organic

Four Science-Backed Benefits To Eating Organic

Organic Foods: What You Need To Know

# 29

# SOURDOUGH BREAD – CRAZY HEALTHY

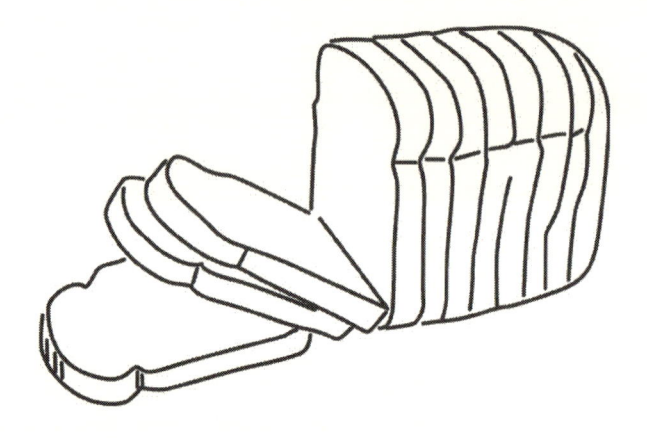

It took me one year to learn how to ferment my own sourdough starter. Was it easy? No. Was it worth it? Yes. I began to understand how truly unhealthy my gut was. Could I get well? At the time, I was 66 years of age and turning 67 (I turned 70 in June 2019). What did I expect and what does healthy feel like? My gluten/grain free diet had worked, and somewhere along the way, I read how functional doctors felt about getting the insides healthy. I decided to do what they recommended.

Functional physicians, that insurance companies do not cover, seem to be on the same page as me. I thought the body could detox in a healthy way and mine did. I read what some doctors said about using foods and infrared saunas to get those metals out of my body, and I did it and was successful. I also thought the body could correct cataracts, which right now is happening (see the Cataracts No More chapter).

I believed that we had become unable to absorb vitamins and minerals through our stomachs and if I wanted to get well I had to work at that too. So what exactly did functional doctors recommend doing? Here is where the sourdough comes in. Sourdough bread is a healing food, so I was forced to learn how to ferment my flours and then produce bread.

Sourdough bread is flour sitting on the kitchen counter for approximately 5 - 7 days. It gets fed like a baby. For gluten free it is fed three times a day and somewhere around the third day bubbles start to form. Those tiny bubbles are what we want to see happening. Those bubbles are called "wild yeast" and have lactobacilli growing. I thought this was a bad thing until I learned that it is a good part of lactic acid. It is friendly bacteria that live in our digestive tract and other parts to the human body. This stuff is so good for us and it is only produced in sourdough bread, fermented vegetables, cured meat, wine, vinegar, and homemade yogurt (not store-bought, sorry).

It was recommended that I soak my grains but that is something I only do for buckwheat breads. I do, however, buy sprouted flours so I am one step ahead of the game without the soaking.

Much discussion has gone on about modern grains and the health issues they produce. I had actually been grain free for three years, but if I ferment, then all of the micronutrients, minerals, and vitamins will go into my body and help me heal. For that reason I no longer purchase store-bought yeasted gluten-free breads. I don't think they are healthy. My breads are made the way nature intended. Fermenting sprouted gluten-free grains like rice, sorghum, and oatmeal and then turning that into sourdough breads is my healthy way to go.

Further Reading

If you are reading the paperback instead of the ebook - you can type each title below in your computer search bar and find the referenced article.

A Healthy Bread That Is Good For You!

5 Reasons To Make Sourdough Bread Your Only Bread

Why Sourdough Bread Is One Of The Healthiest

# 30

# SOY – SO CONFUSING

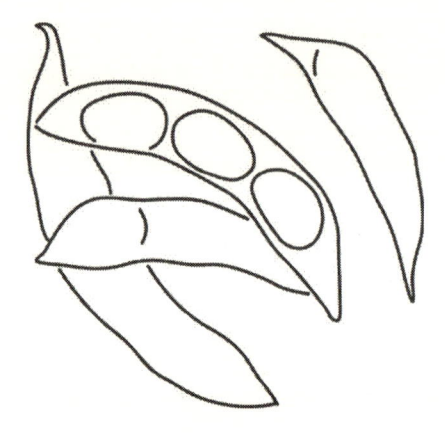

Soy is a confusing substance. The USDA says it's good for us, but I wanted to make sure that I wasn't being misled again. I had been a vegetarian for many years and had been eating it regularly. Now years later I had to really take a hard look at one my favorite go-to foods and the reality of what was sold in the United States. It always starts with the right questions. Why did Asian people benefit so much from soy and here men grow breasts from too much? Why do American women <u>not</u> benefit from what I thought was a miracle food?

As usual, the prompt for my investigation was my food intolerance chart showing soy as mildly reactive (the MRT test I take regularly – see testing list in Chapter 13 – it's the absolute best). Because of that reactivity, I had to find soy in my diet and eliminate it, at least until it turned non-reactive again. I wanted to peel the onion and find out more about it as well.

Here is the low down on soy. Keep in mind this is a food source for vegetarians who think that they are healthier than meat eaters. It is also used as a hidden filler for many fast food restaurants. This is particularly troubling because little children don't know what they are being fed.

Of course I know that in Asia many people eat soy every day and they have lower risk of breast cancers and seem to be healthier and outlive those of us on the Western diet. That is why I thought it was good. Sadly by now you know if I am writing about it, then something isn't kosher.

There are two types of soy - fermented and non-fermented. I ferment almost all of my vegetables, so I know which one I would prefer. Fermentation adds all sorts of health benefits to food. The fermented soy is what is being eaten in Asia, but not here. Even though this country does not understand moderation, it's hard to calculate how much soy you are ingesting, if it's hidden from you. It seems that the American food industry has found a cheap, non-fermented filler, so it's being used in a ton of foods. It's being poured into almost everything including chocolate. Years ago when I was growing up we never saw soy in candy and chocolate.

So what *does* soy do to women? It causes young girls to go into early puberty and raises their sex drive. Like they need to have sex at an earlier age! It also fools around with the endocrine system and can cause infertility in both men and women. This stuff is not sounding so healthy or good for humans. The final straw was when I read about the kind of soy milk or soy products made in our country that cause cancer.

Soy that is not fermented is filled with something called Xenoestrogens. How bad are they? Well you decide after I describe what they do. They are endocrine disrupters and once the body builds up abnormal levels of estrogen produced by this chemical, breast cancer, diabetes, miscarriages, obesity, and sexual issues appear. When you order in a restaurant do you say, "I'll have the soy burger with a side of breast cancer?" I hardly think so.

I also read about something called Hexane and why we should all be concerned about its use in (non-organic) soy processing. This Hexane is one very bad dude as it is a neurotoxic petrochemical solvent that is being used in the processing of all non-organic natural soy products and even some organic. The EPA listed this Hexane as a hazardous air-polluting product, but gives companies the green light to use it on supposedly healthy soy products. Once again I say to myself, "are you kidding me America?" Why would anybody drink soy milk, eat veggie burgers, or anything that contained soy unless it is organic and even then, unless each company was scrutinized? No more soy for me. For soy sauce I now use coconut aminos as an alternative and I'm happy with that. No looking back.

Further Reading

If you are reading the paperback instead of the ebook - you can type each title below in your computer search bar and find the referenced article.

Tempeh Vs Tofu: Which Plant Based Protein Is Healthier?

Fermented Vs Unfermented Soy: Which Is Better?

Xenoestrogens: How To Limit Exposure To Toxins Found In Everyday Products

## 31

# STEVIA – NOT WORTH THE RISK

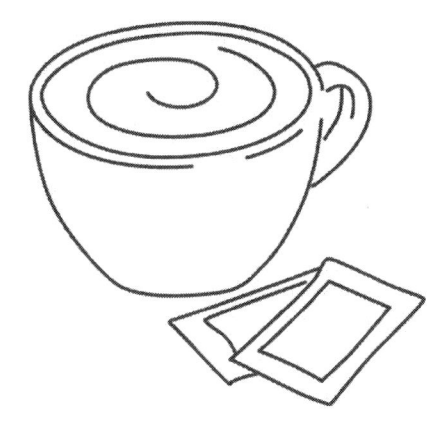

When I was first diagnosed with type 1 diabetes many moons ago, I had to ditch sugar in my coffee and go to a sugar substitute. I started with *Sweet and Low* and called it the pink cancer packet. I hated the taste so I stopped using it and turned to alternatives like honey and maple syrup, which didn't seem to raise my blood sugar as much.

When *Equal* came out I tried using that and called it the brain drain, which I thought produced Alzheimer's. Sometimes I would hold up each packet for my husband and ask, "would you like brain drain or cancer with your muffin this morning?" Of course we laughed but there was a seriousness underlying my question. I realized I was better off with nothing and waited for something better to come on the market.

Along came *Splenda*. I looked for research on it and found nothing, so I called it the "mystery sweetener" and waited for information. When nothing came out I switched to it and used it for many years thinking it was a safe choice.

One day while sitting with a friend's son, who worked in the field of research, I asked about *Splenda* and waited while he cleared his throat and caught his breath. He said it causes gout, tooth decay, heart disease, type 1 diabetes, reduces gut health, makes medication less effective, and when used in baking produces chemicals called chloropropanals. After that I went home and threw out all of my precious *Splenda* and waited once again. Darn it, I hate black coffee.

Then along came *Stevia* and I thought, "natural - how can it be bad? Can this be my solution, once we get used to the taste?" The taste was too much for Larry to get over, so he opted to just use sugar once in awhile, but I kept using *Stevia* while I researched it. Our country calls it the "healthy sweetener" and so did I until I found out the facts.

Stevia can or may alter DNA and chromosomes

It can or may contribute to cancer

I read that if used in moderation *Stevia* might be ok but I chose to stop using it. I turned to my last option, which was *Xyla*, made from birch and not corn. I still use *Xyla*. It claims to have some health benefits, but only time will tell. I have cut my sugar substitution down to "once in a while" and not every day. It wasn't easy but now that I make my own nut milks for my coffee, I stick with those and don't have to reach for an artificial sweetener.

Further Reading

If you are reading the paperback instead of the ebook - you can type each title below in your computer search bar and find the referenced article.

Does Stevia Have Any Side Effects?

What Is Stevia And How Healthy Is It?

# 32

# SUGAR – DANGEROUSLY SWEET

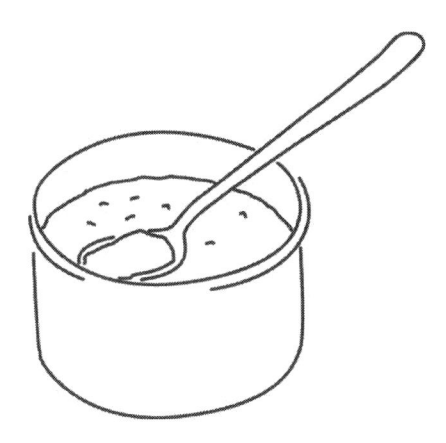

I take the Oxford Bio Medical Technologies MRT test about every six months to a year to evaluate my food intolerances (a simple blood test that shows which foods I eat that I am intolerant to during any given period of time and should not be eating - see Testing section in Chapter 13). The results vary and I may be tolerating a certain food just fine one year, and not tolerating it the next. That is why I like this test so much. I find it helpful, accurate, and a necessity if I want to stay healthy. This test is great to stop the inflammation in our bodies and it's also great for weight loss. The report it generates is essentially the ideal diet for the person who was tested. The program you follow is based on your individual blood test. No one's test is the same and no one's food program is the same. You are an individual with specific needs.

One time a few years ago, my results showed that I could not eat cane sugar. I found this surprising because I generally don't eat anything with cane sugar, or so I thought. That is until I found out that it is in absolutely everything and I have no idea why. It seems that almost every single prepared food contains some form of cane sugar, fructose, maple, and other sugars. I even found cane sugar in nut milks. I decided to see just how many products the public eats every single day that contain some form of sugar. In addition to cold cuts and nut milks, why is cane sugar or any other sugar in tomato sauce?

Why put so much sugar in children's cereals when we all know about weight and diabetes being an issue in our children? What about those "healthy" nut butters /nut milks and the added sugar? Why would McDonalds put sugar in their french fries and all of their rolls? How about their fish and chicken? Why so much sugar in yogurt which renders it unhealthy?

So how bad is sugar for the human body? I knew I had to get it out of all the foods I ate for at least three months to stop my inflammation. This was survival for me. It could be for you too. They even put this stuff in bacon, except the most expensive bacon.

So if companies can leave the sugar out, why do they put it in? One word: addiction. They want you to love the product they sell and what better way then to turn on the good-feeling button. You will go back for more and more and more. It's a strategy that works, but to the detriment of our health.

In 2015 new guidelines were recommended to limit how much added sugar could be put in everyday foods. Without you knowing, big food companies make sure that you eat about 160+ lbs. of this chemical per year (yes it's a chemical). Try lifting 160 lbs. And we thought eating fat was bad. If you want the facts, sugar is far worse than healthy fats, and far worse than too much salt when it comes to disease. Sugar is the main ingredient for very bad health.

Do I use sugar now? Yes, in moderation. Sometimes I want some in my coffee, so I rotate pure maple sugar or dark molasses and now I am trying something new - date sugar and coconut nectar. I don't use it often. I sweeten my baked goods with prunes, apricots, unsweetened applesauce, bananas, and figs. I get a healthy dose of fiber and the fruit binds my gluten-free cookies and gives them the taste of the fruit. The fiber in those fruits stops the sugar spike and instead raises my blood sugar more slowly.

Studies have shown that sugar becomes addictive, just like drugs. The more you eat, the more you want. When you give it up, you actually go through withdrawal.

So why does the United States government allow this horrible product in almost ALL of our food? Here is the truth behind the why. The U.S. government subsidizes corn so high fructose is cheaper than sugar. What the government should do is subsidize healthy food. A candy bar shouldn't be cheaper than an apple.

<u>*The evils of sugar summarized*</u>:
Sugar is a nutritional void with no health benefits

Sugar is fattening and will raise bad cholesterol

Sugar rots our teeth

Fructose, a type of added sugar, can cause non-alcoholic fatty liver disease

Sugar causes the body to have insulin resistance, which causes obesity and type 2 diabetes

Sugar at high levels will cause cancer and if a tumor is present, sugar will feed it and help it grow

Sugar affects the hormones and the chemistry of our brains and we become sugar addicts. You eat it and say yummy in my tummy and then it turns on the endorphins, so you always want more

My interest in this peaked when I had to look for foods without sugar. There turned out to be not enough choices for me. I had to rely on myself once again. If I wanted a safe option for cold cuts I would have to go out and buy my own meat slicer. So I did. I cooked my proteins without the chemicals and then sliced them. I froze each serving in three-ounce portions and took out what I needed the day before. My kitchen was now a deli. A deli without the hotdogs. They all contain sugar.

I cannot tell everyone what to do, but I can suggest you cut out all sugar, fructose, and use real honey in moderation and watch what happens.

Further Reading

If you are reading the paperback instead of the ebook - you can type each title below in your computer search bar and find the referenced article.

This Is What Happens To Your Body When You Eat Sugar

The Sweet Danger Of Sugar

Sugar Subsidies Are Anything But Sweet

Dissecting Girl Scout Thin Mints - It Isn't Pretty

## 33

## TIN FOIL (ISN'T ANYMORE)

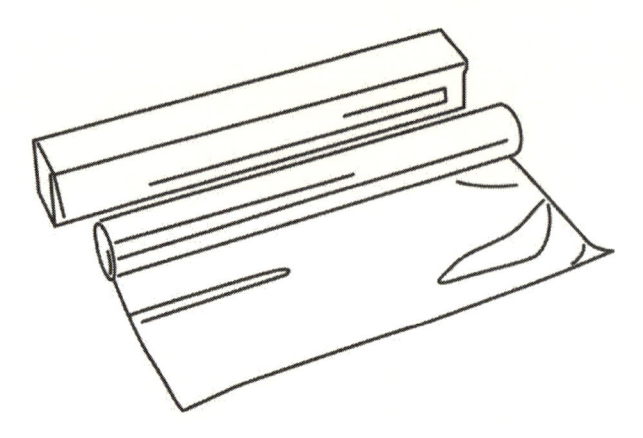

I thought I had the beginnings of Alzheimer's disease several years ago because I became very forgetful. I can't remember exactly when I made the connection (see, forgetful!) between the foil we cook on and wrap food in and my memory issue, but I did. I also didn't know what I could use in place of it, and I had not even looked at the safety of plastic wrap. I had to take on one thing at a time and that particular week I focused on tin foil.

The history of tin foil is really interesting. In 1910 the first aluminum foil plant opened in Switzerland by the Rice Falls. They used the water from the falls for energy. J. G. Neher & Sons owned the company and they produced the first endless rolling system. What I discovered was that tin foil was used to fill cavities prior to the 20th century. I laughed because I used foil to make table decorations and wrap presents when I ran out of wrapping paper. It's so shiny and pretty. So I got the history and found out that tin foil was actually made from tin. Then they changed the recipe and turned tin foil into aluminum foil. Tin is more expensive than aluminum and aluminum is one of the most abundant metals found on earth so for a big corporation it's a no brainer. The bottom line always wins.

When I researched the safety of this substance I found more indecision and each article or doctor said something different. One article said that aluminum has no place in humans and only causes toxicity. So what was I to do? I had to keep investigating. At the end of the day it comes down to how much of it we are ingesting. A little bit won't do harm, but because we get it in drugs, water, some foods, cookware, and deodorant, it becomes a lot more than we bargained for.

I decided to get it out of my diet and found a list of where aluminum is hiding. I also wanted to understand how the body sucked it up. Once I read enough I decided that since no one seemed to know definitively if it was bad for me, I better assume it's *really* bad for me. I took action.

**Deodorant** – I switched to a gluten-free powdered deodorant from Savonnerie called Pit Stop. (www.gfsoap.com) I don't even need it all the time. Since I detoxed my body, I don't smell at all, at least I don't think I do!

**Tin Foil** (which is really aluminum) - I replaced it with brown parchment paper to use when cooking and bought all glass for my oven. Pyrex pin plates have become the center of my universe and brown parchment paper without dyes as well. Glass is cheaper and it's not poison. You have to wash it, but who cares?

**Pans** – I switched to stainless steel and ceramic without the use of aluminum in any products. I bought an amazing and expensive set of pots and pans and they were worth every penny.

I do as much as I can to keep my family safe, but as you are learning from this guide, there is so much that big companies put into our products, it is up to us to decide what we knowingly are willing to ingest or use on a daily basis. We have to pick our poison. And now I never worry about Alzheimer's disease because I dance every day, and dancing keeps that horrible disease at bay. That, I firmly believe.

Further Reading

If you are reading the paperback instead of the ebook - you can type each title below in your computer search bar and find the referenced article.

Why Do We Sometimes Call Aluminum Foil Tin Foil?

High Levels Of Aluminum In 80% Of People Tested For Toxicity

## GAIL KEEHN DVORETZ

### 8 Ways To Protect Yourself From Aluminum Poisoning.

# 34

# WHEAT – NOT THE WAY GRANDMA REMEMBERS IT

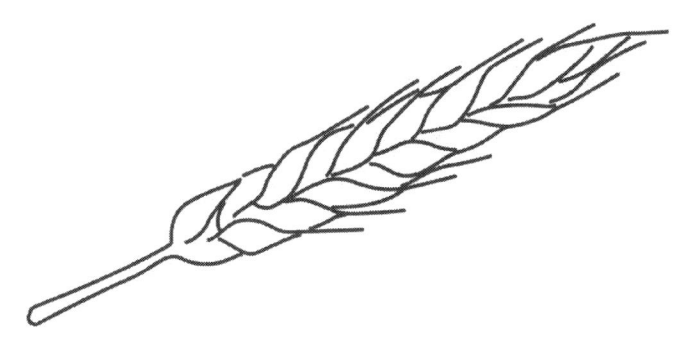

As I write this it's National Pasta Day. Not a day I celebrate at all. Currently across the globe dietary diseases are on the rise and obesity has spiraled out of control in America. Why are so many Americans obese, as in more than 30 lbs. over their ideal weight? Do we really eat that much more than people in other countries or is it <u>what</u> we eat? Could it be both lack of movement and overeating? Or could it be what the food industry is selling to us? Why is there such a big problem and how can we fix it? Can a slight change in diet do the trick?

The problem requires a multi-layered approach, but I think there are things we can do for ourselves right away and when people come to me for help in getting healthy, I start with a few key tips. I let them know up front that exercise is critical and portion control changes everything. The amount of food we see as a portion is skewed. For a visual – you can cut a Cheesecake Factory entrée into thirds to equal one very generous portion. More than that leads to trouble.

One also has to look at the "new" wheat of today and make a decision to cut it out along with other gluten grains. Sugar needs to be a thing of the past and be used only once in a great while. With portion control, wheat, gluten, and sugar elimination, and a little bit of exercise, the rest is just time. Healing the body and the mind takes time. There is no magic pill and there is no quick fix. Period.

So let's unpack the wheat issue further. We touched on it in the gluten chapter. The wheat we eat today, "super wheat," triggers weight gain and disease. Why? I believe it is not just gluten and wheat but the kind of wheat we eat that triggers this chronic disease called obesity. Add in the fructose and other sugars and we now have a sick, overweight America.

All we heard for years from our government was to eat as much healthy wheat as possible and I did. Remember the food pyramid? They said wheat had all the vitamins, minerals, amino, and high fiber necessary for a healthy colon and body. At that time I was a vegetarian and I felt wheat was a safe, healthy food. I ate it almost every single day. I believed the FDA was out to make sure the public knew the facts and I believed they knew what they were doing. I no longer believe that.

The many components of super wheat contribute to both weight gain and to many major diseases. When they spray Round-Up glyphosate on this modified wheat and other grains to speed up growth, it's rendered poisonous. All of the diseases it triggers will kill you no matter how old you are when you get them, or what you do to treat them. You're left with a critical choice. Get off the super wheat like I did or roll the dice. What sacrifices are you willing to make to get fit and stay healthy?

Genetically modified super wheat drives disease because it contains a kind of super gluten with a super starch (amylopectin A) that causes a high level of inflammation. It also contains ingredients that are so addictive; you keep coming back for more and more. Kind of like cigarettes, which we know the FDA finally declared toxic to human beings. They won't come out with such a declaration about wheat just yet. They don't want to lose their moneymaker. But stay tuned, one day it will come out just like it did with cigarettes.

When I used to eat whole wheat bread, my blood sugar would spike up and not come down and that is what it is doing to everyone. When your blood sugar spikes, your body makes a lot of insulin. Insulin is a fat producing hormone, and if you develop insulin resistance, good luck trying to lose weight. The more wheat you eat, the more insulin you make, and the fatter America gets. You might as well eat candy for the same amount of blood sugar spike, and much more satisfaction.

The medical community once again is far behind other countries with regard to gluten intolerance. By the time the medical community in America gets it, millions more will be gluten intolerant and becoming very sickly. People can have gluten insensitivity without celiac disease, so they will get many unnecessary diseases as a result of the inflammation. There are millions of people in America suffering from mystery autoimmune diseases of idiopathic (or unknown) origin. This is not a coincidence. The best, cheapest way to treat these is to eliminate gluten from your diet. No doctor visits and no pills - just a conscious lifestyle choice. Try it for six months and see how you feel. The results will surprise you. It will take years to completely heal, but you'll definitely feel a difference within weeks and months. And the world is much more gluten-free friendly than when I started out in 2009! You can actually eat out in restaurants now without wait staff looking at you like you have three heads when you ask them to wear gloves while handling your plate.

If you have any digestive issues, any allergies or asthma, food intolerances, osteoporosis, chronic fatigue, other autoimmune diseases, or any inflammatory issues like irritable bowl, gallbladder disease, and diabetes, go gluten free and you will feel better. This I know to be fact. I have seen many people over the years do what I did and get well. These are people who felt it was more important to get well than to eat that pasta and bagels. Will I eat that stuff ever again? Absolutely not.

Does this mean that everyone should be gluten free? I am not a medical doctor but for many people I believe going gluten free could start the healing process like it did for Larry, Lannie, and me. I have included the three hundred symptoms of gluten intolerance in the further reading section below, and it is scary. When I give classes, I hand out the sheet with these 300 symptoms listed. Many people check off a number of the same symptoms I had. After the class many people decide to go gluten free and never look back. I hope you'll join us.

Further Reading

If you are reading the paperback instead of the ebook - you can type each title below in your computer search bar and find the referenced article.

300 Signs And Symptoms Of Celiac Disease

Is Wheat A Perfect Chronic Poison?

I Stopped Eating Grains For A Month - Here's What Happened

Why Is Gluten Bad? The Shocking Dangers Of Today's Gluten

GAIL KEEHN DVORETZ

## ARE YOU READY TO DETOX?

### MEDICAL

# 35

# CATARACTS BE GONE!

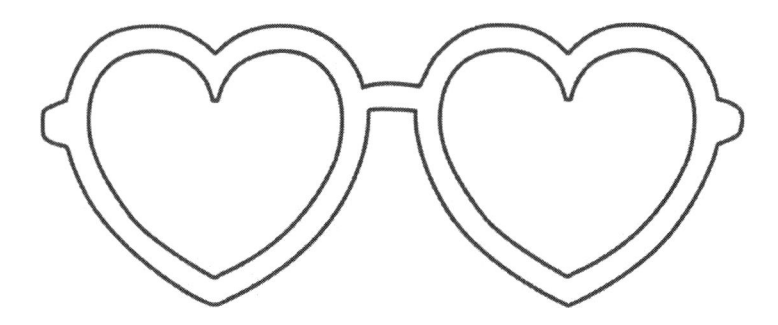

In the summer of 2016 I went from just having cataracts that never progressed from year to year to OMG I am going blind! This all happened in one year and I wanted to know why. What had changed in me? Could it be put into remission or placed on hold until further notice?

First was my blood test for heavy metals. I found out that I had heavy metals in my blood and that could cause cataracts all by themselves. Then I found out that diabetics have a higher risk due to fluctuations in blood sugar and that cannot be helped as I will always be a type 1 diabetic. I could not change the diabetes thing but I could get rid of the heavy metals. What else was I missing and again could my eyes be corrected with anything or was surgery the only possible answer?

I kept on reading and once again I found more information than I bargained for including things I didn't want to know. The title of one article was *"Eye Disease Resulting From Increased Use Of Fluorescent Lighting As A Climate Change Mitigation Strategy"* (read it here). This abstract talked about how the "new" light bulbs were increasing eye disease. What was odd about this was that I had just gotten energy saving lighting. Had these new fluorescent LED lights exacerbated my cataracts? It seemed strange that this had happened within a year of getting the new lights. I also had the heavy metal issue and type 1 diabetes. It was a triple whammy.

What I discovered was that the new lighting increased eye disease by about 12% and that it may be the cause of 3000 cases of cataracts every year, plus another eye disease called Pterygium. Of course I never want to give information out when I only have one abstract but it was certainly something worth looking at. As soon as I showed my husband the information he removed all the new lighting and brought back the old bulbs. Yes, the old bulbs made my room hotter but I didn't care. I was trying to save my eyes and not the world right now. One thing at a time. Is this what had added to my new cataract issue? For someone like me whose first thoughts are with saving our environment, it was an eye opener, (pun intended).

The doctor gave me about three months and said that if I didn't do cataract surgery, I would be blind. Type 1 diabetics avoid surgery like the plague. There are always higher risks and I was scared. I planned my surgery for sometime in July 2016 and then decided to do more research and find some way to put those cataracts to sleep. I was told by three doctors that there was no way that I could prevent my eyes from getting worse, but I always feel it is important to find out what other parts of the world might be using to fix cataracts. I found a treatment in the form of eye drops.

I decided to find out more about these drops and when I had read enough to make an educated decision, I called my doctor and spoke to my compounding pharmacist. He explained that he had another patient who was older than me and didn't want the cut and paste cataract surgery. She had gone for the same drops as me. She never went back for surgery, so I decided to have them made up and give them a try. That was three years ago.

When I went back to my eye doctor for another exam he seemed uneasy. I told him what I had been putting into my eyes with great results. I knew I could see again and could drive at night without fear. I told him if I were in his shoes I would let patients who are just diagnosed with cataracts go on these drops to prevent surgery. Surprise, surprise, he said he couldn't do that. Why could he not do that? I did it and had successfully avoided surgery. I was getting glasses in 2017 when he said in 2016 that he could not correct my vision with glasses anymore. What more proof did he need? First I was blind and then I wasn't. I could not understand why a doctor who takes an oath to do no harm would not share my eye drops with people who would need surgery if they didn't do what I had done. So now once again I get to share this information with as many people as possible.

Here is the prescription. In a nutshell I was already taking a powdered form of the stuff I put into my eyes but I was taking it to get my body healthy. Who knew that a year later I would be using it to keep my eyesight.

1.25% GLUTATHIONE
1.25% ABSORBIC ACID

6.25% DSMO

NAC that I purchased on Amazon as a separate drop

Put all this into an eyedropper to be taken three times a day into clean eyes and made by a trustworthy compounding pharmacy. The DSMO transports the medicine into the cells to make them healthy again.

Recently I added Dexterity Health Liquid MSM with Vitamin C and NAC Drops Advanced Antioxidant Eye Drops

So far so good and I am now wearing my new glasses. Do I know if this will work forever? No, I don't. But I am willing to try and think outside the box, which it seems doctors are not willing to do. I also take Camu powder, which is very high in Vitamin C, and Glutamine in my morning drink. This is kind of like what I am taking in my eyes. What I started doing to heal my gut is now helping my vision.

I also wear special glasses when working on my computer. The light coming out of this technology will cause harm to your eyes as well. These glasses can be bought on Amazon and are called UVEX Skyper Blue Light Blocking Computer Glasses. These are not the only ones that are sold, so research and see what is good for you.

I read that many physicians knew about the eyes not doing well with the new LED lights and went out to purchase as much of the old lighting as possible for themselves. I have also purchased enough of the old incandescent lights to last us throughout our lives, like the smart doctors did.

Further Reading

If you are reading the paperback instead of the ebook - you can type each title below in your computer search bar and find the referenced article.

Why Light Bulb Choices Matter

The Dark Side Of LED Light Bulbs

Cataracts - The Options

# 36

# STATINS – NOT THE ONLY OPTION

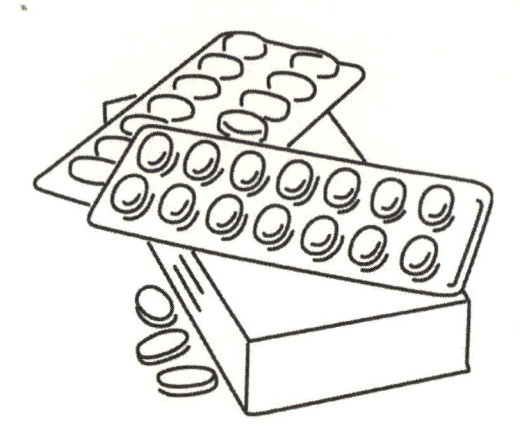

As soon as a doctor sees cholesterol over 200 they start talking statins. My first experience with a doctor who wanted me on statins happened when I was 61 and ended up in a hospital with a potential problem. I had a death in my family that caused anxiety, but it seemed like a heart attack. As soon as you get to the hospital and they think you are having heart issues, they want to slap a nitroglycerin patch on your arm. When I asked what the patch was for, the nurse said it was protocol for people having heart issues. I refused the patch and told her that until I am diagnosed with a heart attack, she should hold on to her patch filled with nasty drugs. I said no to this nurse a lot. The following day I met the heart specialist and without the doctor even examining me, he told me to go on statins. When I asked why he listed his reasons.

I was over sixty
I was American
I was a type 1 diabetic
My cholesterol was 224

I laughed and told him that my triglycerides were 48 and my HDL was 101. Whenever you have that high an HDL, your LDL's will also be higher and so will all the other test numbers. He didn't agree with my decision about the drugs and then suggested that I have an angiogram done immediately because of his concerns. I told him I would think about it but would need to talk to my endocrinologist. Sadly Dr. Carrington said that as a diabetic I should have it done, and then we could make a decision about doing anything else.

When the specialist came back the next day we talked about my "A" particles and the fact that the test I take for cholesterol showed my ratio for having a heart attack at less than two, very low. He looked confused about the new test I had been taking for two years. I was having the particles that run through my arteries tested. You see I don't take the useless tests that most doctors prescribe their patients. I use a more in-depth and thorough blood test that gives much more information about the subject's heart health. I said I would take the test but I would bet him his salary that my arteries would be clear. He didn't agree with me. I told him we would wait and see. I made him promise that if I was right, he would give patients my test and read up on all the bad things about statins. If I was wrong, I would take them. But I wasn't worried. I knew I was right.

The next day I was taken into the surgical unit where my test was done in really pretty colors and I sang to everyone in the surgical room. When I woke up I asked my questions…stents or no stents? New arteries or could I keep the ones I had? When I was really awake I asked for the surgeon and his partner laughed. He had left and taken his checkbook with him. This doctor said I had pristine arteries and neither one could figure out how this was even possible. How could a 61 year old, brittle type 1 diabetic born and raised in America have clean arteries? I left the hospital the next day and refused the statins.

It turned out that although my cholesterol was around 224, I had all "A" type particles, the type of cholesterol that took good stuff through the arteries on fluffy clouds. This good stuff didn't cause heart attacks and cleaned out the arteries unlike the "B" small particles that were bad. So I went home to learn more about heart health and statins.

First I discovered that statins are drugs that doctors recommend for all diabetics as protocol and you know what I think of protocol for all. When you take statins, the good cholesterol is removed along with the bad in your arteries and brain. So now years later the true facts about those drugs are coming out and it is scary. The FDA has now stated that a warning should be added to those drugs stating that statins will increase the risk for both diabetes and loss of memory. If the FDA wants a warning label, imagine how bad it must be. New research is divided. Some say they do more harm than good and some say just the opposite. I also wonder who is doing the latest research. I have learned that the companies that sell these products do the research and that, dear reader, is a bald-faced conflict of interest.

> Here are the harmful statin facts:
> memory loss
> diabetes risk increases
> muscle pain
> hemorrhagic stroke
> myopathy also known as muscle weakness
> elevated liver enzymes

I feel there are better ways to get that cholesterol down and one way is to just exercise. Exercise can turn the bad "B" particles into good "A" ones. Exercise also helps lower the bad levels. Eat more healthy foods that are high in fiber like beans, oats, fruits, and vegetables (organic of course). Limit foods high in saturated fats and increase foods high in omega 3s. I eat salmon, sardines, halibut, and trout. These are the good fish that lower your cholesterol instead of raising it. You can also choose meat lower in fat and cook it in a crockpot with vegetables. You can take red yeast rice. You can also try citrus bergamot, which has been hailed as an all-natural statin. Monitor your results carefully. It is important to understand the drugs that are prescribed to you. I never just take something unless I get the facts about the product, and you shouldn't either.

Quest has a new test called Cardio IQ. This is what everyone should be taking and learning to interpret the test.

## Further Reading

If you are reading the paperback instead of the ebook - you can type each title below in your computer search bar and find the referenced article.

Citrus Bergamot: The All Natural Statin?

Side Effects Of Statins

Is It Time To Retire Cholesterol Tests?

## 37

# THERMOGRAPHY VS MAMMOGRAPHY

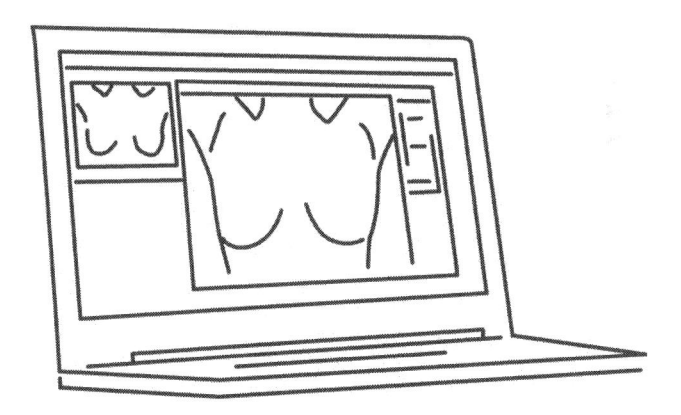

In 2014 I started reading about what causes all kinds of cancers and what showed up was my yearly mammogram. Again I sat there perplexed thinking, "Why would I be doing something yearly to prevent breast cancer when the thing I was doing could cause this cancer?" Don't doctors know what I was reading? I called my sister Lannie and told her what I had a just learned and explained that I was never going to have a mammogram ever again. I would find something to replace that with and get back to her.

Our grandmother had breast cancer but she also smoked three packs of cigarettes a day. She had her yearly mammogram and yet the test didn't detect the tumor until it was too late. So the test still isn't perfect if you have dense breasts, which I do. Now I had to find a substitute without the radiation. I felt this was going to be hard and I was hoping that I could find something viable. Three weeks of research later I found something called thermography.

After reading all I could about thermography, I discovered that my insurance company would not cover this non-invasive, no radiation, and chemical-free diagnostic exam. I decided to read more about it. It seemed like something I could use to help detect breast cancer but I would still need something more because just using heat sensors might not be enough. I opted for thermography with an ultrasound. The jury is still out about thermography but it is out about mammograms as well.

There are conflicting stories about everything we use and that is why I am always researching. I did discover that a combination approach to breast health might be the safest way to go. This can include breast exam by an OBGYN, breast self-examination, thermography, MRI, and an ultrasound at the hospital. Just because I choose breast exam yearly by my OB-GYN, and thermography with ultrasound doesn't mean I am right. It is what I am choosing to use for me. I just don't feel comfortable submitting to something every year (mammogram) that might cause the disease I am trying *not* to get. You may feel that mammography is the best screening tool. Like everything else in this guide, it's a personal decision, I just want to educate and present options.

Further Reading

If you are reading the paperback instead of the ebook - you can type each title below in your computer search bar and find the referenced article.

4 Breast Cancer Screening Tests You Should Know About

Breast Thermography: What You Need To Know

Comparing Mammography And Thermography

# 38

# VITAMINS – HERE'S THE SCOOP

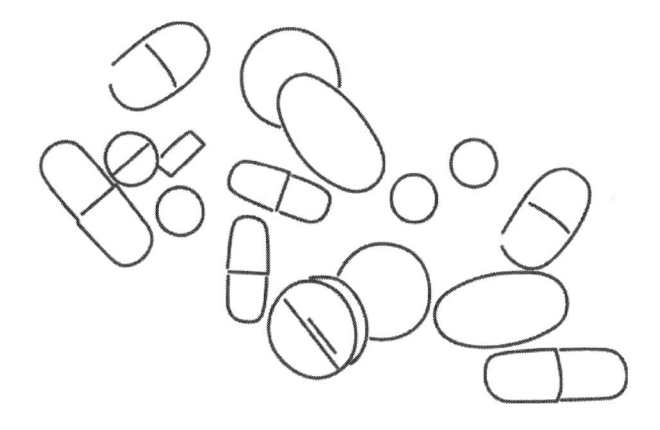

Just when I think I get it right I find out that I got it wrong. This has happened several times along my health journey. A perfect example is with vitamins. When I took a test some time ago, I found out that I needed to get more vitamins and aminos in my body. I needed selenium and pantothenic acid. I also needed calcium. I thought I would just go to the local store and pick it up. It seemed easy enough. Everyone buys their vitamins from either Costco or BJ's because they are cheaper. I was using an online company because it was easier to buy online, as I was still sick. But now, in my life, I have to research which vitamins contain corn, wheat, dairy products, and possibly chemicals. This would entail reading the back of every pill container to find the one I could take. I didn't think that a vitamin pill would contain anything but the necessary vitamins I needed right? Wrong.

Early in the morning, which is when I do all my research because the phone isn't ringing, I got out my computer and sat on the couch to begin my search. After about three hours of looking, I got up and wanted to throw myself out my window. Finding gluten-free, corn-free, and dairy-free vitamins was going to be impossible. And then I found something I knew nothing about, magnesium stearates. I thought, "well I don't want magnesium in my pill, I just want calcium with boron and maybe some other things that help my bones stay strong." So I looked up magnesium stearates and my hair stood up on end. I knew I had to find a vitamin pill without magnesium stearates at all costs. I marched into my bathroom closet and turned around all the vitamins I had been using from a company I won't mention and there on the back of each pill container was listed magnesium stearates.

Well you might ask what is so bad about magnesium and that is what I thought until I kept reading. Magnesium stearate is a white powdery substance that they use to lubricate our vitamins so they don't stick together and slide down the big machine and then fall in the bottle. This saves them money but does nothing for your health or mine. Well, still not so bad right? Big deal I thought, until I read a story about our inability to absorb this stuff. So I decided to do a kitchen experiment to separate fact from fiction.

I took out three water glasses all freshly cleaned and began with three types of vitamin powders. One vitamin I found <u>without</u> magnesium stearate and one with it. I threw a tablespoon of the powdered product in and it went bye-bye. I put the vitamin with gelatin and it went away pretty quickly. The one with the magnesium stearates just sat there, as it would sit in your stomach making toxic waste with very little absorption. I was so angry that I called the vitamin company that I had been using and told them what I had discovered. They got very quiet because they knew. I told them I was returning all my family's vitamins for a full refund and that they had better refund my money and they did.

While looking for a safe product I found two companies that don't use any chemical fillers or magnesium stearates – Dr. Ron's (www.DrRons.com) and Dr. Mercola (www.DrMercola.com). I refer to them often in this guide. When I found Dr. Ron's site, he had an article about the use of stearates in vitamins! My eyes widened and I knew it was fate. Yes, I probably pay more for my products, but why buy something your body isn't going to absorb?

It occurred to me that no wonder I was lacking in vitamins even though I took so many. Non-absorption was the culprit. Most of the stearates come from China and are full of cottonseed oil, and the crops in China are massively sprayed with horrible chemicals. It's a recipe for disaster for someone like me. The more I read about how contaminated our vitamins were, the angrier I became. I now call any vitamin company I might use to ask about the extra ingredients in their products. They are required to tell you.

<u>Further Reading</u>

If you are reading the paperback instead of the ebook - you can type each title below in your computer search bar and find the referenced article.

Wondering Why It's Important To Choose A Magnesium Stearate Free Brand?

Magnesium Stearate - What Is It?

5 Dangerous Ingredients In Your Vitamins And Dietary Supplements

# AFTERWORD

I hope that in the previous pages you have learned something new and have hope, whatever you may be facing. As I mentioned in the Preface, I didn't add my partial autobiography for any other reason than to perhaps identify a link between my life experiences and my health. My journey to stay alive and healthy has been exhausting but I realized that I could share this information so someone like me could benefit from it. That thought made my journey worthwhile.

Even through all of the horrible experiences I've had in my life, beginning in childhood, I won the lottery a couple of times. In many ways, I was lucky. I've compared myself to a cat with nine lives. I always manage to take bad things and turn them into good things.

How many people can live on the street, survive, and afterwards be taken in by a family willing to shelter and nurture?

How many people can barely read in 11th grade and still get a college education with the help of intelligence and determination?

How many people can almost die from the flu and blood sugars reaching 900 and turn that into a journey toward good health?

How many people can beat fibromyalgia, chronic fatigue syndrome, alopecia, and 39 medications and turn those into a life full of vitality and joy?

How many people can take up dancing as a hobby and become a ZUMBA® instructor at 69 years of age?

Against all odds I am still here and I am still dancing. I learn new things every day and I still face challenges, but I keep researching. I keep finding new products and new methods to deal with whatever comes along. Just because life dealt me a bad hand didn't mean I had to settle for it. I dealt myself a different hand and moved forward. I encourage you to do the same. I now have a busy, happy, and healthy life and I am motivated every day to teach others how to get and stay healthy. That is why I wrote this book.

If you are interested in seeing some of the new products I discover or new treatments, please follow me on social media. Gluten Free Gail rose from the ashes in 2009, and she's here to spread knowledge and give encouragement! I am very active on Facebook and Instagram, as well as my website www.GlutenFreeGail.com, and if you find something new you'd like to share, please do so.

We're all in this together, and despite the fact that our government and our health care system don't always do the right thing, we don't have to be led like lambs to the slaughter. We can fight back. Knowledge is power and the truth is out there.

If you take just some of this book and use it I will have done my job. I will have made my donation to our world. Believe You Can And You Will. I'm going to include that in huge letters on the next page so you'll always remember. Believe in yourself and know that I believe in you.

# BELIEVE YOU CAN AND YOU WILL!!!

# SHOPPING

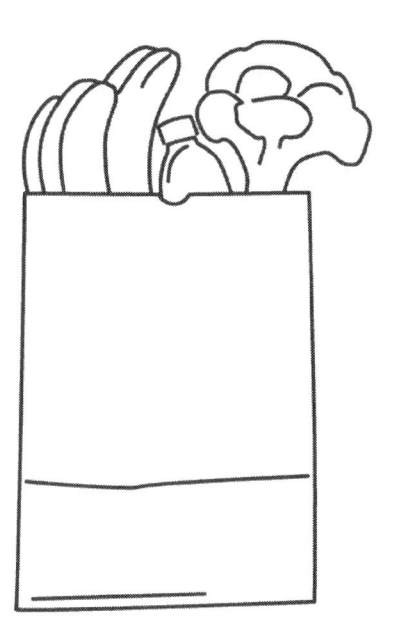

I take my shopping, cooking, and eating very seriously. If a company isn't willing to speak with me and assure me that their products contain no dangerous ingredients, I won't go near them. I am constantly on the lookout for new, safe, and delicious gluten free and healthy options to make life a little easier and a lot more delicious. Over the years and through much trial and error, I have found products that I am proud to recommend. I am happy to say that the list is growing almost weekly.

### *Amazon.com*

Amazon is a great company and continues to carry many foods that are both healthy and gluten free. For gluten free just type the words in the search bar and their gluten-free options will come up. I also buy my organic bean pastas and Numi Tea from Amazon.

### *www.ThriveMarket.com*

Thrive Market often has lower prices on many organic and gluten-free foods. They also have unusual types of foods and things that cannot be bought at stores or at other online markets. They do charge a fee every year to belong but they save both time and money in travel time to hunt down groceries. They have better products and prices. I often purchase my soaps and shampoos at this site.

### *WildernessFamilyNaturals.com*

I buy my nuts from them as they are raw and I can get sprouted flours as well.

### *Nuts.com*

I buy nuts, flours, and dried fruits from this site. They also have jellies and other items that are gluten free.

### *WiseChoiceMarket.com*

This company will deliver many of the things that I make myself. I cook a lot but sometimes I'm tired and I also have friends and clients who do not have the time to make their own healthy foods. This is my go-to-site. They will deliver healthy foods without GMOs. They have a large collection of Paleo-, WAPF- (Caveman Diet), and GAPS- (diet that heals leaky gut, anxiety and other inflammatory issues) friendly foods. You can purchase raw cheese, soaked nut butters, fermented vegetables, or organic bone broths, and wild seafood. This is a great site.

### *BlueMountainOrganics.com*

I purchase organic raw sprouted nuts from this company. The taste of these nuts is so different. Once you are used to them you will never go back.

## *BarryFarm.com*

Thanks to Barry Farm I was able to produce bread products using flours no one had ever heard of ten years ago. They saved me from starving when I went gluten free. Back then there were no other companies selling unusual flours. I learned how to ferment buckwheat from their products and produce bread when I was not able to eat much of anything else. They label everything that is gluten free and then have recipes that help understand how to use a new grain or flour. Examples of their flours are garbanzo bean, black bean, plantain, green pea (which I love baking with), and sorghum. They also sell beans, dried fruit, spices, nuts, and seeds. They are reasonably priced.

## *HealthyFlour.com*

This company is called To Your Health Sprouted Flour Co. I buy most of my flours from them as they have explained where they get their rice. I want my rice flour and all other flours without the arsenic, thank you very much. The flours are also sprouted which is more readily absorbable. They have 32 gluten free products to choose from and I made an amazing sourdough sorghum bread using their products. Their flours always seem to ferment the best.

## *www.DrRons.com*

I purchase almost all of my vitamins from Dr. Ron. Dr. Ron passed away in 2017, but before that, he would call you back if you had questions!

## *VitalChoice.com*

I buy all my fish, both canned and frozen, and most of my meat from Vital Choice. I try to purchase once a month and always look at their bonus each week to determine when I will make a purchase. If you spend a certain amount of money you can get fish, vitamins, organic fruit, or meats. They are not cheap but you will get the best products.

## ***What's In My Kitchen?***

I am constantly discovering new products, but you will frequently see the products listed below in my cabinets and fridge, if you ever find yourself in my kitchen. To stay updated with all the new products I find, follow me on facebook at Gluten Free Gail (https://www.facebook.com/GlutenFreeGail), Instagram (https://www.instagram.com/glutenfreestairwaytohealth), or visit my website, www.GlutenFreeGail.com. Rest assured that I ALWAYS test out the products I recommend. I have tasted dozens of horrible products so you don't have to! What I recommend below is guaranteed delicious.

### *Sweet Things*

**Wedderspoon Gold:** 100% Raw Manuka Honey in glass jars only. This company also makes

**Honey Lozenges**: Lemon Bee Propolis and one with Ginger and Echinacea and an active honey level of 15 plus. www.Wedderspoon.com

**Organic Coconut Nectar**: I get mine at www.ThriveMarket.com

**Vanilla Frosting:** Simple Mills Organic Vanilla Frosting. This is available at Whole Foods and through www.Amazon.com. www.SimpleMills.com

**Sugar:** Biona Organic Rapadura, I get mine at www.Amazon.com

**Sugar:** Alter Eco Organic Mascobado Cane Sugar, I get mine at www.Amazon.com

**Sugar:** Big Tree Farms Organic Coconut Sugar Blonde, I get mine at www.Amazon.com. You can also check out their site, www.BigTreeFarms.com

**Beet Sugar:** Real Foods Beet Sugar is for people who are allergic to coconut or honey. It is great for baking and available at www.Amazon.com

**Xylitol**: This is a sweetener made from birch. I use it when I am going to make a cookie or cake. As a diabetic, I have to watch my intake of carbs with sugar. I do not recommend sugar substitutes unless it is a special occasion and someone with diabetes is also eating my deserts. You can get this at www.Amazon.com or www.ThriveMarket.com.

**Pure Date Syrup Organic and Gluten Free:** Date Lady brand. You can buy online directly from this company at www.ILoveDateLady.com

**Chocolate Syrup:** I use Wildly Organic. This product is delicious and makes an amazing hot chocolate! www.WildernessFamilyNaturals.com

**Buckwheat Honey**: A very good and healthy brand I use is from

Sandt's. You can buy this product at www.Amazon.com and read about all of their honeys at www.SandtsHoney.com. This product has high anti-oxidant compounds and macronutrients.

**Chocolate**: We like Enjoy Life chocolate, 69% cacao dark. You can get it at www.ThriveMarket.com and check out their other products at www.EnjoyLifeFoods.com. I also use Pascha chocolate chips which I get at Whole Foods or www.ThriveMarket.com. Check out their other products at www.PaschaChocolate.com.

**Money on Honey:** Delicious sweet chocolate bars available at www.Amazon.com or at https://www.drogachocolates.com/collections/put-your-money-on-honey.

**Primal Kitchen**: Dark Chocolate Almond Collagen ProteinBar. These are delicious and healthy. Get them at Publix, Whole Foods, or online at www.PrimalKitchen.com.

**Jennies**: Absolutely yummy chocolate macaroons. Paleo, gluten free, dairy free. I got them at Publix, or you can get them at www.JenniesMacaroons.com.

## *Breads*

I often make my own breads and like to experiment with different gluten-free flours, but not everyone can do that. Here are some options for quick and delicious gluten-free bread.

**Against The Grain:** These rolls are my favorite. They get crispy when toasted and make an amazing egg sandwich. www.AgainstTheGrainGourmet.com

**Udi's**: Udi's makes the best gluten-free English muffins around. www.UdisGlutenFree.com

**Chebe**: These bread mixes are easy to prepare and come in interesting flavors. This company also makes pizza crusts. You can buy the mixes on www.Amazon.com or directly from www.Chebe.com. Whole Foods sells their frozen dough.

## *Spices*

**Spicely**: Organic spices that I order directly at www.Spicely.com. They can also be found at some Whole Foods stores.

**Simply Organic**: These organic spices can be found at Whole Foods or online at www.SimplyOrganic.com.

**Frontier Spices**: Organic only and I can purchase them from the company online at www.FrontierCoop.com or at Whole foods.

**McCormicks**: These are the only company's spices that I will use if I cannot find organic. Available at all grocery stores.

## *Extracts*

**Nielsen-Massey:** Pure orange and vanilla must be purchased online at www.Amazon.com and you can read about the company and all of their products at www.NielsenMassey.com.

**Simply Organic:** Madagascar pure vanilla can be purchased at Whole Foods or online at www.SimplyOrganic.com.

### *Oils*
**Publix Green Wise:** Organic virgin coconut oil unrefined

**Nutiva**: Organic shortening containing palm oil and coconut oil (I have some issues about using palm oil because it is hurting our environment). You can purchase these products at www.ThriveMarket.com and read about their company and products at www.Nutiva.com

**Field Day:** Organic extra virgin olive oil. You can order it at www.Amazon.com and read about their company and other products at www.FieldDayProducts.com

**Chosen Foods:** Avocado oil you can purchase at www.Amazon.com, www.ThriveMarket.com, as well as many other online retailers. Read about their company at www.ChosenFoods.com.

**Spectrum Naturals:** Organic sunflower oil. This can be purchased online at www.Amazon.com or www.ThriveMarket.com

## *Cheese*
Raw, organic, and grass fed – only from my local farmer's market.

## *Chips and Snacks*

**Jacksons Honest:** Sweet potato chips. These are available at www.ThriveMarket.com, www.Amazon.com, www.VitaCost.com, or at their site, www.JacksonsHonest.com.

**Let's Do Organic:** Toasted coconut flakes unsweetened. You can get them at Fresh Market, Whole Foods, or online at http://www.edwardandsons.com/ldo_info.itml.

**Jica Chips:** Different flavored jicama chips available at www.JicaChips.com.

**Harvest Snaps:** SnapPea crisps are available at most grocery stores and online at www.Amazon.com, www.ThriveMarket.com, or at their website www.HarvestSnaps.com.

**Tropee**: Dried fruit bars from Colombia. They are delicious and available to buy at www.Amazon.com.

**Bare:** Organic apple chips and coconut chips. These are available at www.Amazon.com or at their site, www.BareSnacks.com.

**Barnana:** Chewy banana bites available at www.Amazon.com. You can snack on them or use them as breading for chicken and fish. They have many other delicious products at www.Barnana.com.

**Kind:** These bars are available in many flavors and they have a new flavor, Pineapple/Banana/Kale/Spinach that is great for you and delicious. You can find Kind bars anywhere. www.KindSnacks.com.

**Flackers:** Organic flax seed crackers with rosemary (very strong rosemary flavor). They have other flavors as well. I eat flax seeds in moderation because of their heavy levels of cadmium. You can get them at www.ThriveMarket.com, www.Amazon.com, or at their company site, www.DrInTheKitchen.com.

**Mary's Gone Crackers:** Also contain flax seeds and available in different flavors. You can get them at www.ThriveMarket.com or at their site www.MarysGoneCrackers.com.

**Inka Chips:** Plantain Chips available at www.ThriveMarket.com or www.InkaCrops.com. I usually make my own but these taste good and when I am in a hurry they are a great snack to take with me.

**Kettle Brand**: Organic potato chips can be found in most grocery stores and online at www.Amazon.com, many other online retailers, and at their site, www.KettleBrand.com.

**Go Raw**: This company has ginger snaps and many other products available at their website, www.GoRaw.com or at www.ThriveMarket.com, or www.Amazon.com.

**Stretch Island**: These organic fruit snacks are great for kids. They are available at all grocery stores and you can read about the company and their products at www.StretchIslandFruit.com.

**Newman's Own**: Organic prunes. Prunes are dried plums and plums need to be organic. They are on the dirty dozen list almost every year! Newman's Own products are available in every grocery store in America.

**Wellsley Farms**: Organic raisins. Raisins should always be bought organic as they are dried grapes, and grapes are always on the dirty dozen list. You can buy this product at www.Amazon.com, www.bjs.com, or at www.ThriveMarket.com.

**Mariani**: Organic sun dried unsulfured calimyrna figs. You can get these at www.Amazon.com or www.bjs.com. They are great to use for jams and cookie stuffings. You can put these figs or prunes in a food processor and voila.

**Lundberg Sweet Dreams:** Organic dark chocolate rice grain cookies. Lundberg is the only company whose white rice I will use as they test for heavy metals and are completely honest about which products to avoid if you have problem. I know this because I called them and they explained everything to me. This is a great company with great products available at www.Lundberg.com.

**Glicks:** These are coconut macaroons for the Jewish holidays and can be bought throughout the year at Whole Foods and www.Amazon.com.

**Nuts:** I only eat organic nuts from www.Nuts.com or www.WildernessFamilyNaturals.com.

## *Tomato Sauces*

You should always purchase in your tomato sauce in a jar. The only exception is a company called POMI (www.pomi.us.com). They sell a single serve box container and they now have organic products. I know that my grocery store carries it but you have to check with your local stores and request that they carry POMI as well.

**Bionaturae Organic Tomato Paste:** This paste is no salt added and I get it from www.ThriveMarket.com.

**Flora:** Organic italian strained tomatoes, also available at www.ThriveMarket.com. www.FloraFoods.com.

**Jovial:** Organic diced tomatoes that can be purchased at Whole Foods. www.JovialFoods.com.

**OrganicVille:** Organic tomato sauce with basil. This can be bought at Walmart, Target, or from www.Amazon.com. www.OrganicVilleFoods.com.

### *Syrups, Jellies, Spreads, Mayonnaise, Mustard, Ketchups*

**Eden:** Organic apple butter and organic applesauce that I get at www.ThriveMarket.com. I use applesauce in place of eggs for baking. www.EdenFoods.com.

**Wellsley Farms:** Organic pure maple syrup. You can buy this product at www.Amazon.com, www.bjs.com, or at www.ThriveMarket.com.

**Fiordifrutta:** Organic fruit spread with no corn of any kind in it. They have all sorts of spreads. Some of our favorites are strawberry and blueberry. Make sure to refrigerate after opening. I buy these at Whole Foods or at Walmart. www.fiordifrutta.it.

**Nocciolata:** Organic hazelnut spread with cocoa and milk. They also have a dairy-free product. You can get it at www.Amazon.com. www.NocciolataUSA.com.

**Artisana Organics:** Raw tahini sesame seed butter and raw coconut cocoa bliss. I purchase these from www.ThriveMarket.com. They have a whole line of organic nut butters. www.ArtisanaOrganics.com.

**Primal Kitchen:** Mayo with avocado oil. This can be purchased at Publix or online at www.ThriveMarket.com. It took me years to find a mayonnaise without soy or other bad things, so I love this product. It contains avocado oil, eggs, organic vinegar, sea salt, and rosemary extract. This product is made the way people use to make their own years ago. www.PrimalKitchen.com.

**Follow Your Heart:** Soy-free vegenaise mayo. I buy this at Whole Foods when I don't want eggs in my food. You can also get it at www.Amazon.com. www.FollowYourHeart.com.

**Vermont Village:** Spiced apple butter. This is great on everything including pancakes. I also put it on toast so I don't have to use butter. It's available at www.Amazon.com. www.VermontVillage.com.

### *Pasta and Rice*

Rice is of concern to me because brown rice contains arsenic. I don't serve rice often in our home, but when I do, I buy white rice.

**Lundberg:** California white jasmine or basmati. You can get it at www.Amazon.com or www.ThriveMarket.com. www.Lundberg.com. I also like to buy basmati from India as this rice also has low levels of arsenic.

**Lotus Foods:** This company is wonderful. They state that none of the regions where Lotus Foods rice is grown have any known arsenic contamination. I get this at www.Amazon.com. www.LotusFoods.com.

**Explore Cuisine:** Organic edamame and mung bean fettuccine, organic black bean spaghetti and organic adzuki bean spaghetti. You cannot beat these pastas for people with blood sugar issues. You can get these products at Publix or online at www.ThriveMarket.com. www.ExploreCuisine.com.

**King Soba:** Organic buckwheat noodles. Buckwheat is not made from wheat. It is actually a fruit seed in the same family as rhubarb so it is safe for people with celiac disease or someone with gluten intolerance. You can buy them at www.Amazon.com or www.ThriveMarket.com. www.KingSoba.com.

**Andean Dream:** Quinoa pasta. This pasta is both organic and corn free. It is available at Whole Foods and online at www.Amazon.com. www.AndeanDream.com.

When you want to dine out – check out www.FindMeGlutenFree.com for gluten free dining near you.

## *Healthy Makeup Choices*

**Red Apple Lipsticks**

www.RedAppleLipsticks.com
They say all their products are gluten free.

### Ecco Bella
www.EccoBella.com
They say their products are gluten free as well as chemical free and vegan.

### Vapour Organic Beauty
www.VapourBeauty.com
No chemicals, organic, and vegan.

### Bare Minerals
www.BareMinerals.com
They cannot guarantee gluten free although they say most of their products are. Because I avoid all gluten, I won't use them.

### After Glow Cosmetics
www.AfterGlowCosmetics.com
First gluten free certified makeup line - also organic, and vegan.

### ZuZu Luxe
www.GabrielCosmeticsInc.com
I buy this line at Whole Foods and I love it!

### Joelle Cosmetics
www.MyMineralGlitters.com
This company has a gluten-free line. They are also corn free, soy free, and casein free.

### Monave Mineral Makeup
www.Monave.com
Organic, gluten free, and 95% vegan

# RECIPES

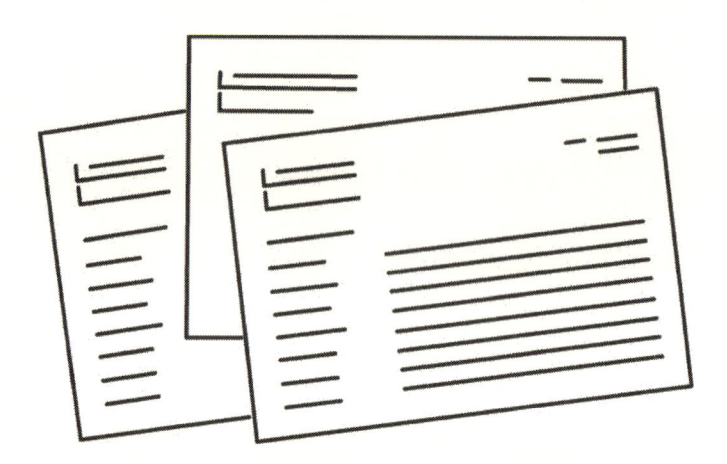

I have dozens of recipes that I have tested out over the years. I am always searching for quality ingredients, (see shopping section), and experimenting. I wanted to include some of the dishes that were a "home run" in this book so you have the option of trying out some amazing food as you venture into your new lifestyle. The recipes I've included are healthy, easy to prepare, and delicious. Enjoy! And please check out my website (www.GlutenFreeGail.com) and my Instagram page (Gluten Free Gail Instagram) for more. I post new recipes and meal ideas daily on my Instagram page.

## Shrimp Scampi

Peel and de-vein 1 lb. of extra-large shrimp. Make sure you get either wild-caught or farm-raised in the US – all other farm-raised fish around the globe are toxic.

1 lb should be enough for three people
1 cup of butter (I use goat butter)
¼ cup olive oil
4 cloves minced fresh garlic
1 tbsp organic fresh parsley (chopped)
2 tbsp rice flour or breadcrumbs
3 tbsp brandy
Organic lemon to taste
Extra whole garlic cloves (optional)

Melt the butter and mix with the olive oil
Put garlic in and stir
Mix in the brandy

Throw the shrimp into the sauce and stir.
Make sure there is enough sauce to go around for all of the shrimp.
If you want more sauce go ahead and mix some extra together.
Put all of this into a glass baking dish making sure that each shrimp is laying flat.
Spread the breadcrumbs and the parsley
Squeeze lemon on the shrimp to taste
Bake at 425° for 20 minutes – then put under the broiler to crisp the top, watching it to make sure it doesn't burn.

## Chicken Loaf

12.5 oz. of Harvest Creek organic canned chicken
1 organic egg
2 cups of chopped up fresh organic spinach
Salt to taste

Spray a glass baking dish with olive oil spray and put all ingredients in
Bake at 350° for one hour
This chicken loaf is baked and has only three ingredients
Easy to make and delicious

## French Onion Soup

Prepare Bone Broth - Organic grass-fed bones about 2 pounds with some meat on them. Place them in a crockpot with distilled water and two tablespoons of apple cider vinegar. Add one onion with the skin and any other spices you like and let it cook on high for one hour. Turn it down to low for 48-72 hours then turn it off. Once it is cooked, drain it and get rid of the vegetables. Many people use the bones for a second cooking because the bones are so expensive. I put my broth in small containers so I can put in the refrigerator right away. You don't want to cool it on a counter. You can also buy grass-fed broth frozen at Whole Foods.

Cut up four large onions and sauté them butter or olive oil. Make sure the onions become caramelized. They need to cook about thirty minutes.

Combine the onions with the homemade beef broth, throw in a little red wine, cook about 15 more minuets on the stovetop-and you have French onion soup.

Option: serve in small bowls with a crostini, add cheese, and broil in the oven.

## Roasted Eggplant With Goat Cheese, Onion, Tomato, And Spinach

2 organic eggplants
2 organic onions
2 organic tomatoes
2 slices of goat cheese
1 cup fresh spinach

Place parchment paper on a baking pan and spray olive oil – spread onion and eggplant (spray olive oil on top of vegetables as well) and cook at 400° until caramelized

Layer eggplant with goat cheese, onion, tomato, and spinach
Cover with more parchment paper and tin foil on top to melt the cheese

Serve and enjoy!

## Crustless Baked Quiche

8 eggs
¼ cup Ripple plant based milk
½ cup caramelized onions
1 cup raw organic spinach
Salt and Pepper to taste
Cayenne pepper to taste

Mix all ingredients in a bowl
Coat a round glass pie plate with spray oil (olive or avocado)
Bake at 350° until done
Put in the broiler to brown the top, but keep an eye on it as it browns quickly

This is great for brunch when company is coming

## Flour-Free Crockpot Roast

4-5 lb chuck roast
1 large onion chopped
4 cloves of garlic
2 celery stalks chopped
4 carrots chopped
4 cubes of homemade beef broth or you can buy bone broth at a store
(If you buy it add 1/4 cup or more)
1 cup of red wine and 1 cup of water or two cups of water if you don't want to add wine
4 tbsp Nature's Way Always Liquid Premium Coconut Savory Garlic Oil

Sear the roast either in a pan or in your crockpot. Add coconut garlic oil to the crockpot or pan. Sear the roast on all sides in the garlic oil. This can take about 5 minutes on all sides. Make it crispy for maximum flavor and remember it will get soft in the crockpot.

Remove the seared roast, add the onions, and cook for a few minutes until slightly brown. Then add all the other chopped up vegetables and let them cook for about 15 minutes to give them flavor.

Put the roast back in the slow cooker and add the liquids. Cover and cook on high one hour and then lower for another 8 hours.

If you want to thicken the gravy bring it to a boil and stir in three tablespoons of arrowroot and stir while it thickens.
Flour free thickeners don't fare well on the second go around so use it all up the first night you serve it.

You can always serve the gravy on the side.

## Rice Casserole

3 cups white rice
2 eggs beaten
10 oz. bag of organic frozen cooked kale
½ cup or more (if needed to thicken) nutritional yeast
1 cup of caramelized onion (pan fry with oil of your choice)
Fresh garlic or garlic powder to taste
Stir all together
Feel free to add any other spices you might like
Prepare a casserole dish with spray oil, add mixture, and bake at 350° for 40 minutes

GAIL KEEHN DVORETZ

**Gluten-Free Stir-Fry**

Cook your gluten free rice noodles ahead of time
Stir-fry bok choy, scallions, green onions, red onions, carrots, spinach
Add fresh garlic, coconut aminos*, and olive oil to these organic vegetables
When the vegetables are cooked, throw in your pre-cooked rice noodles
Add chicken soup and any other spices you might want
Easy and delicious!

*A gluten-free alternative to soy sauce

## Gluten-Free Rice Stuffing

One package of rice cakes soaked in water
Cook one cup of white rice and drain
Place rice bread in the oven and let it bake for one hour at 225°
Cook 1 onion, 3 stalks of celery, and fresh garlic chopped up in olive oil
When that mixture is golden put it into the stuffing mixture
Stir those together
You can throw in nuts, sunflower seeds, or pine nuts. Just make sure you roast them in the oven for 10 minutes

Spray a glass casserole dish with olive oil and put the stuffing into it
Bake for 15 minutes at 350°
Use veggie broth or turkey bone broth to keep it moist - about 3 cups stirred in before baking

**Vegan Sushi**

Onion
Avocado
Asparagus
Cucumber
Carrots
Peppers
2 cups of sushi rice (it needs to be sticky)
Nori sheets can be bought at Whole Foods or online
Shred vegetables

Cook rice but add 3 tbsp of rice wine vinegar to the water when cooking the rice
Put the nori dry side up and spread rice on it
Add mayonnaise (optional) then add the vegetables and roll
Slice on an angle, plate and be proud!

**Gluten-Free Macaroni And Cheese**

24 oz. of rice pasta uncooked
3 cups of milk
3 cans evaporated milk
½ cup butter
¾ cup cream cheese
4 cups shredded cheddar cheese
1 cup shredded Swiss cheese
Black pepper and salt to taste

Put uncooked pasta in a large crockpot

Melt all the milk and cheeses in a separate pot stirring constantly so it's creamy

Pour cheesy mixture all over the pasta

Closed the crockpot up and cook for about two hours

Add more milk if it starts to dry up

This is not to be considered low anything - but it is gluten free and easy.

**Vegetarian Gluten-Free Pasta**

Store-bought gluten-free pasta of your choice (see shopping list for suggestions)
Spinach
Tomatoes
Mushrooms
Onions
Fresh parmesan cheese
Homemade tomato sauce (organic tomatoes, garlic, onions, salt, pepper, oregano in a vita mix and it's done)

*For a non-vegetarian protein option, add clams on top

## Three Ingredient Oatmeal Crackers

3 cups of oatmeal flour or any other gluten-free flour
Mix it with water and olive oil until it has the consistency of pancake mix

Spray parchment paper with oil on a baking tray and spread the mixture out flat

Bake at 350° for 20 minutes on one side and when you can flip it with a spatula (and it doesn't stick), go ahead and flip it and bake the other side for 20 minutes

You can also cut with kitchen shears into cracker size at this point before they completely crisp up

Watch them carefully and take them out one at a time when they are crispy enough

## Gluten-Free Coconut Egg Bagels

½ cup coconut flour
½ tbsp baking powder
½ tsp baking soda
2 cups cashew cheese or mozzarella cheese
2 tbsp coconut oil or butter
3 organic eggs

Preheat your oven to 400°
Mix all dry ingredients together
In a separate bowl, mix all wet
Make sure to melt the cheese
This dough will be sticky
You could always add in another egg or more oil if the dough is too dry

Break into four pieces and form into a bagel
Place on brown parchment paper make sure you put a hole in the middle
Bake for around 13 to 16 minutes
These bagels should be golden

Once cooked, slice and freeze so they will last longer

## Gluten-Free Irish Soda Bread

2 cups of rice flour
One egg beaten
1 ½ tsp baking soda
1 tsp baking powder
½ tsp guar gum
¼ cup sugar (I used xylitol)
¾ cup organic raisins
3 tbsp melted butter

1 cup of buttermilk


Preheat oven 350°
Rub oil on a cookie sheet
Put all dry ingredients into bowl, including raisins and stir
In a separate bowl beat butter sugar and eggs until fluffy

Stir together the dry and wet ingredients


Place the flour on a board and knead about 5 times
Place the dough on a cookie sheet and cut into 8 servings but don't go all the way down


Spray oil on top and sprinkle cinnamon

Bake at 350° for 30 minutes
Remove and let cool before slicing


Put parchment paper between each slice and freeze

## Fermented Buckwheat Bread

Ferment 2 cups of buckwheat grounds for 24 hours
You can get them at www.nuts.com
Drain them without washing
Put them in a food processor with 1/2 cup of water and a pinch of salt
Rub oil on a glass loaf pan and then put the buckwheat in
I put it outside on my table where it is really warm (we live in Florida) and left it there for another 24 hours
Make sure it has risen enough to bake

Bake at 350° for one hour and 30 minutes
This is a delicious high fiber bread
Slice and put parchment paper between each piece

Freeze for extended use

**Gluten-Free Bread**

4 cups gluten-free rice flour
2 tbsp psyllium husk
¼ cup applesauce (make your own in a Vitamix!)
1 tsp baking powder
1/2 tsp baking soda mixed in with 1 tablespoon lemon juice – it will fizz
½ cup egg whites
2 tbsp olive oil
Water (as much as needed to make a wet batter)

Put parchment paper into a loaf pan and spray with olive oil
Bake in a preheated 350° oven until done

I test my breads with the meat thermometer - it should read 180
Let the bread cool and then remove the parchment paper and put the bread on a cooling rack

It is the best bread ever

## Coconut Bread

1 cup organic coconut flour
3 eggs
Lemon zest
½ cup desiccated organic coconut
½ cup coconut syrup or sugar
1 cup coconut milk or yogurt
¼ tsp salt
1 tbsp baking soda
1 pinch of cream of tartar
1 cup organic applesauce (make your own in a Vitamix!)
¼ cup organic coconut oil
½ tsp vanilla
¼ tsp cinnamon
If mixture too dry, add more coconut milk
Preheat oven to 350°
Grease a mini loaf tin
Combine the flour, lemon zest, coconut, and cinnamon
Add eggs, combine
Add salt, vanilla, baking soda and cream of tartar, combine
Spoon mixture into oiled tin
Bake for 35 minutes
Cover with foil and bake for another 20 minutes
If still soft in the middle, keep it covered and cook for another 10 minutes
Make sure it doesn't burn
Remove from the oven and allow it to cool slightly before flipping it onto a cooling tray
Leave to cool completely before cutting into thick slices
Great toasted with butter

## Oatmeal Bread

2¾ cups oatmeal flour
½ cup maple syrup or honey
¼ tsp gar gum
¾ cup homemade cashew nut milk
Two eggs room temperature
½ tsp of salt
½ tsp baking powder
¼ tsp baking soda
1 tbsp apple cider vinegar
Stir it all up
You can always add more milk if it's not a banana bread consistency

Spray parchment paper with oil and pour the mixture into a loaf pan
Bake at 300° for one and a half hours
Using a meat thermometer - make sure the bread internally is at 200°

**Cauliflower Crust**

6 cups boiled cauliflower rice (I get mine from Trader Joe's)
Drain the cauliflower until almost dry
Ring it out in a dry towel
This is the hardest part
Make sure it is also completely cool

<u>Make flax eggs</u>
2 tablespoons flax
6 tablespoons water
Stir then let it sit until it becomes gel
Add 3 tbsp nutritional yeast
Mix all three things together and add whatever spices you like
Mix in 1 tbsp of arrowroot or potato starch
1/4 tsp salt
Add the cauliflower

Place parchment paper on a baking sheet
Throw some arrowroot or rice flour on the parchment paper and then spread the cauliflower crust on top - spreading with a fork as thin as you like your crust.
Bake for 50 minutes at 375°.
(Flip after 40 minutes and then finish the last 10 minutes).

Add toppings - any vegetable and any sauce you like works but easy on the sauce because it makes it soggy if too much is added. When all your toppings are on – bake another 15 minutes or until it's cooked to your liking.

## Chia Flatbread Pizza

2 ¼ cups rolled flat oats (I have to use gluten-free oats)
¼ cup chia seeds
3 cups purified water
1 ¼ tbsp baking powder
4 tbsp olive oil
A pinch of salt and some pepper
Mix the chia and oats in 3 cups of water and let them set for 24 hours

The next morning stir your oatmeal and chia then add the salt, baking powder, olive oil and stir again.

Preheat your oven to 400° and spray three glass pie plates with olive oil
Pour the mixture into each pie plate and flatten it so it's thin
I use round parchment paper but you can use just the glass pie plate

Bake for about 25 minutes
I flip mine over to make sure it's golden on both sides
Once out of the oven, put them on cooling racks

Voila! Gluten-free high-fiber pizza crust!

## Cashew Milk

Organic homemade nut milks are so easy to make - and they leave out the toxic carrageenan and gums. They are inexpensive, organic, delicious, and super healthy!

Heat up hot water and let the cashews soak for at least 15 minutes
Add the nuts to the blender with four large dates (no pits)
Add in sweetener, vanilla, cinnamon, ginger or cardamom for flavor
Put it in a glass jar store in refrigerator and use within three days

**Walnut Milk**

1 cup of water (more if you want it less creamy)
½ cup of organic walnuts soaked for 24 to 48 hours
3 dates for sweetness (no pits)
Cinnamon to taste
½ teaspoon of vanilla

Put in blender or Vitamix and blend until creamy
Refrigerate and use within 5 days

**Pistachio Nut Milk**

1 cup of water (more if you want it less creamy)
½ cup soaked organic pistachios (soak for 48 hours)
3 organic dates (no pits)
Blend in the Vitamix until creamy
Refrigerate and enjoy
Sugar-free
Chemical-free
Dairy-free

**Sunflower Seed Milk**

Put one cup of organic sunflower seeds in a glass bowl and fill it with water
Add 2 tbsp apple cider vinegar and cover it with a cloth. Let it sit on your counter for at least 12 hours
The next morning rinse the seeds
Put one cup of seeds in a blender with 3 cups of water or less water if you like it creamier
Place in a Ninja bullet, Vitamix, or any blender and blend on high until you don't see any seeds left
At this point you strain the product if you need to
You can add any type of sweetener you like, vanilla, or even cinnamon

## Kimchi

Fermenting is great for your gut. You can buy fermentation lids for wide mouth mason jars on Amazon and that makes the process so easy.

For kimchi:
Cabbage
Onions
Red hot pepper
Paprika
Cayenne Pepper
Garlic

Put all the spices at the bottom of your mason jar (amounts added according to taste – some people like really spicy, some more mild)
Put in the cabbage, onions, and peppers
In a separate cup mix distilled water with 1 tbsp of salt and stir until dissolved
Add the distilled water mixture to the jar but not to the top, leave 1 inch, keep mixing if you need more liquid
Cover with the fermentation lid and leave out at room temperature for about a week – but check on it on day four just in case
When the fermentation is complete, eat, enjoy, and store in the refrigerator

## Cashew Caesar Salad

For the salad use organic romaine lettuce
Organic strawberries
Roasted organic Brussels sprouts
Add sunflower seeds or any other protein you wish

<u>Cashew Caesar Dressing</u>
½ cup raw cashews
½ cup water
1 heaping tbsp of cilantro or coriander
1 clove garlic
¼ cup olive oil
1 tbsp lemon juice
Blend in Vitamix or blender

**Cashew Dressing**

1 cup of cashews soaked (4-6 hours)
Add ½ cup water
2 tbsp olive oil
2 tbsp organic lemon juice
Chopped green onions to taste
Salt and pepper to taste
Nutritional yeast to taste
Onion powder to taste
Garlic powder to taste
Lemon shavings (optional)

Blend in Vitamix or blender - great with any salad

**Egg-Free/Dairy-Free Mayo**

1/2 cup of avocado oil
1/4 cup full fat coconut milk
1 avocado
2 tbsp lemon
2 tbsp mustard
½ tsp salt
¼ tsp pepper
¼ tsp garlic

Add all ingredients except the oil to the food processor using pulse
Once combined, using high speed on the food processor, VERY slowly add the oil, one small drip at a time, it can take 10 minutes to add the oil

This mayonnaise can last anywhere from 5 to 10 days in the refrigerator, but you'll use it all up before then, it's so delicious

**Super Simple Salad**

Organic mixed greens
Fermented red pepper (you can make this yourself)
Baked salmon
Caramelized onion
Raw onion
For breakfast, lunch, or dinner – this is delicious

<u>Homemade salad dressing</u>:
Leftover fermented brine
Olive oil
Fresh garlic
Dill
Parsley
Mustard
Sweetener of choice

Refrigerate dressing when not using
Take it out of the refrigerator an hour before using again.

## Fermented Vegetable Slaw

Organic vegetables (try Brussels sprouts and carrots)
Slice them up and put them in a glass jar
Add a cup of distilled water
1 tbsp of a really good salt (like Real Salt)
Make the water/salt mixture as many times as you need to fill the jar leaving room an inch from the top

Seal the jars up (you can get the lids at Amazon.com – just look for "fermenting jar lids")
Wait for the veggies to ferment – it will take about 3-5 days

Add nuts for more crunch and a homemade dressing - healthy and really delicious

**Asian Cabbage Slaw**

Thinly slice up a head of cabbage
Chop up any vegetables you want to add to the slaw

<u>Dressing:</u>

¼ cup coconut aminos
¼ cup lemon juice
¼ cup sesame oil
2 tbsp grated ginger
2 tbsp date sugar
2 tsp sesame seeds
¼ cup mayo
2 tbsp apple cider vinegar
Salt and pepper to taste

**Detoxing Cabbage Soup**

1 head of purple cabbage
Water is the base
3 sautéed organic onions
Fresh garlic
Organic string beans
Organic carrots
Organic spinach

Cook the cabbage, onions, garlic, string beans, and carrots in water for about an hour until the vegetables soften. Then add the spinach and let that cook for about five minutes.

Ready to serve, and a great way to detox and lose weight!

## Clam Chowder

Use lobster shells to make a broth
Sauté onion, celery, garlic and some organic ham until the ham is crunchy and the vegetables soft

Sprinkle 6 tbsp of rice flour all over the vegetables and stir
Add the broth from the lobster and cook until thickened

Add sliced potatoes and cook the entire dish for 20 minutes
Once the potatoes are done, put in 24 oz. of clams

Serve and enjoy

**Stuffed Cabbage**

Filling:
1 pound of grass-fed organic beef
¾ cup brown long grain rice
1 onion with 4 cloves of garlic sautéed
1 bag of spinach cooked
1 small whole cabbage that has been put into a pot and steamed for about 10 minutes
Mix every ingredient together except the cabbage

Drain the cabbage and peel whole leaves off
Use about ¼ cup or more of the filling mixture - put inside a cabbage leaf and roll it up
Lay filled leaves seam side down in your pan

Add about ¾ cup of cabbage water into the pan (or tomato sauce)
Lay extra pieces of cabbage on top and cover with parchment paper and tinfoil
Preheat the oven to 350° and cook for 90 minutes

You can then take the cooked stuffed cabbage and brown it on the stovetop with olive oil for color

## Vegan Gluten-Free Sweet Potato Casserole

4 lbs sweet potatoes
4 tbsp coconut butter
1 tsp cinnamon
½ tsp vanilla (optional)
¾ cup Ripple Pea milk
¼ cup coconut sugar
Dash of salt

Mash up the potatoes once they are cooked and mix in all other ingredients
Place in a 2 quart glass casserole dish with pecan topping

<u>Pecan topping</u>
4 tbsp coconut butter
1/3 cup coconut sugar
1/2 tsp cinnamon and nutmeg
1/2 cup pecans chopped
Mix together and place on top of casserole
Bake at 350° for 20 minutes

When the casserole is done and you're ready to eat, place 2 cups of marshmallows on the casserole and broil until they are golden. Leave the oven door open and watch the marshmallows so they don't burn.

## Banana Cashew Cookies

1 cup organic cashew nut butter
2 mashed bananas
1 egg
¾ cup chia
2 tbsp sweetener
¾ cup dark chocolate chips
Mix everything together but put the chips in last
Put the mixture in the refrigerator for 30 minutes
This allows the mixture to thicken
Add more chia if it is not thick enough
Put it back in the refrigerator to allow it to thicken
This could take another 15 minutes

Remove from the refrigerator and make cookie rounds on parchment paper
Use a fork to smash them down
Preheat oven to 350°
Bake for 15 to 20 minutes

These are gluten-free, dairy-free, grain-free, paleo

## Homemade Chocolate

Melt 3 bags of Pascha dark chocolate chips and Enjoy Life organic dark chocolate
Chop up organic walnuts, cranberries, and raisins
Chop up orange peel and coconut chips
Add the walnuts, cranberries, and raisins to the melted chocolate
Add the orange peel and coconut
Spray oil on parchment paper, pour chocolate mixture and refrigerate for three hours to harden

A delicious gluten-free dessert

## Gluten-Free Flan

¾ cup white sugar
2 egg yolks
6 egg whites
½ tsp vanilla
Pinch of salt
1 14 oz. can condensed coconut cream
1 ¾ cups water

Preheat your oven 350°
In a pan stir the sugar on medium until golden
Take a round glass pie-baking dish and pour the sugar in swirling it around so it covers the bottom

In a bowl beat eggs, egg whites, water, condensed coconut cream, vanilla, and salt until creamy
Pour this mixture on top of the caramelized sugar
Fill a roasting pan with hot water halfway up and place a rack inside of that
Put your flan on top of the rack and put into the oven
Make sure your oven is preheated and bake about one hour
It will still be somewhat "jiggly" when it is finished
Remove the pie plate and put it on a rack to cool for an hour
Put it in the refrigerator overnight and serve the next day

Carefully serve the flan from the pie plate – the trick is to get it out without it falling apart
Run a knife around the edge of the pie dish and then turn over onto a plate

## Pumpkin Seed Yogurt

Soak 2 ¼ cup organic raw pumpkin seeds overnight
Pour into your blender with enough water to make yogurt consistency
Add contents of mega flora probiotic pill
Place it in a glass jar, cover it, and put it in the refrigerator for one week

Billions and billions of probiotics
No chemicals, no toxins, no sugar
This is gluten-free, vegan, paleo, dairy-free

## Coconut Fermented Cream Cheese

This coconut cream tastes like real cream cheese
1 can organic heavy coconut cream – be sure to shake
1 glass jar
1 mega flora probiotic pill opened up and put inside the jar with the coconut cream
Stir with a wooden spoon, cover with a cloth, and place on the kitchen counter for three days to ferment
After three days cover and place in the refrigerator and don't taste for another two days
It will taste creamy and tart and will be full of probiotics

## Homemade Apple Juice, Hold The Arsenic

In a Vitamix combine:
2 organic apples cut up with the skins left on
Water
Cinnamon (to taste)
Lemon juice (to taste)
Mix until well combined
Use a nut bag to strain
Pour strained juice into a glass and enjoy

Safe and delicious

## Gluten-Free Donuts

½ cup nut butter (I made my own cashew nut butter)
One medium banana mashed
1 egg
1/8 cup maple syrup
1/8 tsp cinnamon
1 tbsp coconut flour
¼ tsp apple cider vinegar
¼ cup wild blueberries or blueberries
¼ tsp baking soda

Mix the nut butter, syrup, egg, and banana, until they're all combined
Mix everything else together and throw in the blueberries last
I bought a donut pan on Amazon and that's what I used to make these, but you can also use a muffin pan

Bake at 350° for 30 minutes and then check on them – every oven is different so use the toothpick method to make sure they are cooked

## Banana Apricot Chia Bar

3 organic bananas
8 oz. dried organic apricots
10 organic figs
½ cup organic hemp seeds
2 tbsp chia mixed into 6 tbsp water to form an "egg"(wait 15 minutes for the gel to form)

Preheat oven to 350°
Mix all ingredients in a food processor
Spray coconut oil on parchment paper and spread the mixture
Cook for 15 minutes then cool in the freezer until hardened
Cut into squares or bars and put in a container

You can leave them in the freezer or the refrigerator

## Coconut Crème Brulee

1 cup coconut milk
1 cup heavy cream
1 tsp cinnamon
1 tsp vanilla
4 extra large eggs
7 tbsp of sugar (I use coconut sugar)

Preheat oven to 325°
Combine the coconut milk and cream in a pot and bring to a boil
In a separate bowl beat the egg, the cinnamon, the vanilla, and the sugar
***Slowly*** pour the cream mixture into the beaten eggs

Take out ramekins and spray them with coconut oil
Fill them about ¾ full with the egg mixture
Put them in a baking dish and fill the baking dish with hot water
Bake for about 20 minutes until set
If they don't seem set (toothpick test), cook them for another 10 minutes

I eat them warm but my family likes them after they have been chilled

## Coconut Peanut Butter Cookies

½ cup of coconut flour
½ cup of coconut sugar
½ cup of coconut oil
4 organic eggs beaten
2 cups organic crunchy peanut butter
¼ cup organic carrot powder
Add cinnamon or 1 tbsp vanilla if desired
Beat all ingredients together in one bowl

Using a scooper, scoop up a tablespoon
Use your hands to make a ball and place on a cookie sheet or brown parchment paper
Flatten cookie with the back of a fork

Preheat oven to 325°
Bake for 12-15 minutes
You can eat them right away or let them cool
These are a soft batch cookie
I like all of my gluten-free cookies frozen, so after I let them cool, I place them in a plastic bag and put them in the freezer

## Pineapple Upside-Down Cake

2/3 cup coconut flour
½ cup goat butter
8 eggs
¼ cup coconut sugar or sugar of choice
1/8 tsp salt
1 tsp baking soda
1/8 tsp cream of tartar
¼ tsp potato starch or tapioca starch
Juice from canned pineapple
If you need more to thicken batter use full fat coconut milk
1 fresh pineapple sliced (rounds or bite size pieces)
Toasted coconut
½ tsp more of coconut sugar

Preheat oven to 325°
Prepare a pan with coconut oil or oil of choice
Melt the butter, mix with sugar, and blend
Beat the eggs and add to the wet ingredients but temper the eggs first by adding a little at a time…this prevents cooking the eggs when adding them to the melted butter
In another bowl mix the dry ingredients
Now add all the wet to the dry and see if you need to add pineapple juice to produce a batter
This should be sticky and you should not be able to pour it
Spray the cake pan with coconut oil and place the pineapple pieces on the bottom with the toasted coconut pieces and optional added sugar
Pour the batter over the pineapple and coconut
Smooth the bottom with a knife

Cook for about 40 minutes (use the toothpick test to check)
When it is done let it cool and loosen it with a knife
Turn it upside down on a plate and enjoy

## Gluten, Dairy, And Flour-Free Fudge Cake

1 ½ cup organic heavy coconut cream
1 can organic condensed coconut milk
1 tsp Nielsen Massey pure orange extract
2 9 oz. bags of Enjoy Life dark chocolate morsels (they are dairy free)
You can add coconut chips or nuts but it's not necessary

Heat the coconut cream with the coconut milk until it begins to boil
Let it cool for about one minute
Melt the chocolate chips in a microwave bowl
Mix the two together until the mixture is creamy and smooth
Add the orange extract
Stir the mixture slowly to temper it
Spray a glass baking dish (9x11) with coconut oil

Pour the mixture into the glass baking dish, cover with plastic wrap, and place in the refrigerator
It will be ready to serve in about three hours
Store it in a glass container with a tight fitting lid
It will last about two weeks

**Dairy-Free Chocolate Pudding**

3 large avocados really soft and ripe
2 tbsp of honey or sugar
½ tsp cinnamon
¼ cup coconut sugar
6 tbsp coconut cream
2 tsp of coconut oil

Mix it all up in a blender and then put into a small bowl with fresh or frozen berries

## Buckwheat Muffins With Carob Frosting

1 cup buckwheat flour
4 tsp baking soda
½ tsp cream of tartar
1 ½ tsp cinnamon
1 tbsp psyllium husk
4 eggs
3 tbsp honey or blackstrap molasses (diabetic version use xylitol)
7 large organic strawberries or 1 cup berry of choice
1 large banana
Oil of choice to grease the muffin pan

Preheat oven to 350°
Bake for 15 minutes until done
Let cool

<u>Frosting</u>
Mix ½ cup carob powder
¼ cup sugar of choice
3 tbps coconut oil
Add organic sweetened condensed coconut milk or cream (to make it extra creamy)
Mix until it's the desired creamy consistency
Spread on cooled muffins

## Gluten/Grain-Free Banana Bread

2 cups of organic green banana flour
2 tsp of bicarbonate soda
2/3 cup of milk (I use goat's milk because I can digest it better)
½ cup sugar
4 eggs
4 slightly over-ripe mashed bananas
1 cup melted goat butter (or butter of choice)
You can add cinnamon or any other spice of choice
I have added chocolate chips and nuts
Put all ingredients in a large bowl and mash everything together (or use a food processor) until it becomes a pourable batter
It should be relatively smooth

Preheat oven to 325°
Prepare a glass bread pan with oil spray of choice or butter
Pour the batter in and smooth the top
Bake around 35-40 minutes or until done (use toothpick test)
Make sure you put the tooth pick into the center of the loaf
Let it cool on the counter and enjoy

Store the leftovers in the refrigerator or freezer
Gluten-free products often preserve better in the freezer

# ABOUT THE AUTHOR

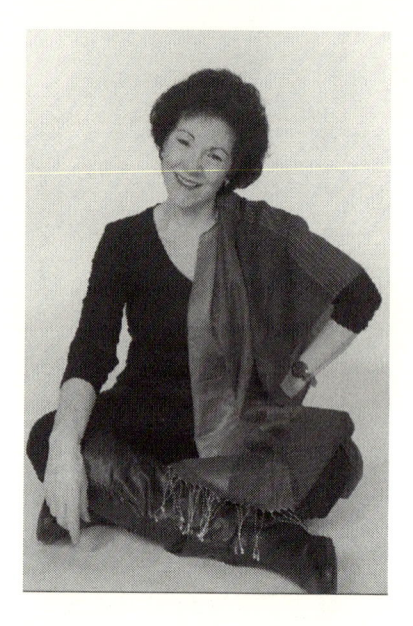

Gail Jacalyn Keehn Dvoretz was a highly regarded special education teacher in Broward County Florida for three decades. She currently works as a state licensed mediator, ZUMBA® instructor, and health coach. She is a mom, wife, sister, grandmother, friend, and community leader. She is also a passionate health advocate who knows first hand that commitment and persistence overcome obstacles. With **Believe You Can & You Will**, she hopes to share her experiences and educate all Americans who are coping with diabetes, autoimmune diseases, and gluten intolerance. **Believe You Can & You Will** is for anyone who has been thrown a curve ball (or ten) by life, has had to be a health advocate for themselves or someone they love, and has wondered what would happen if they simply refused to give up.

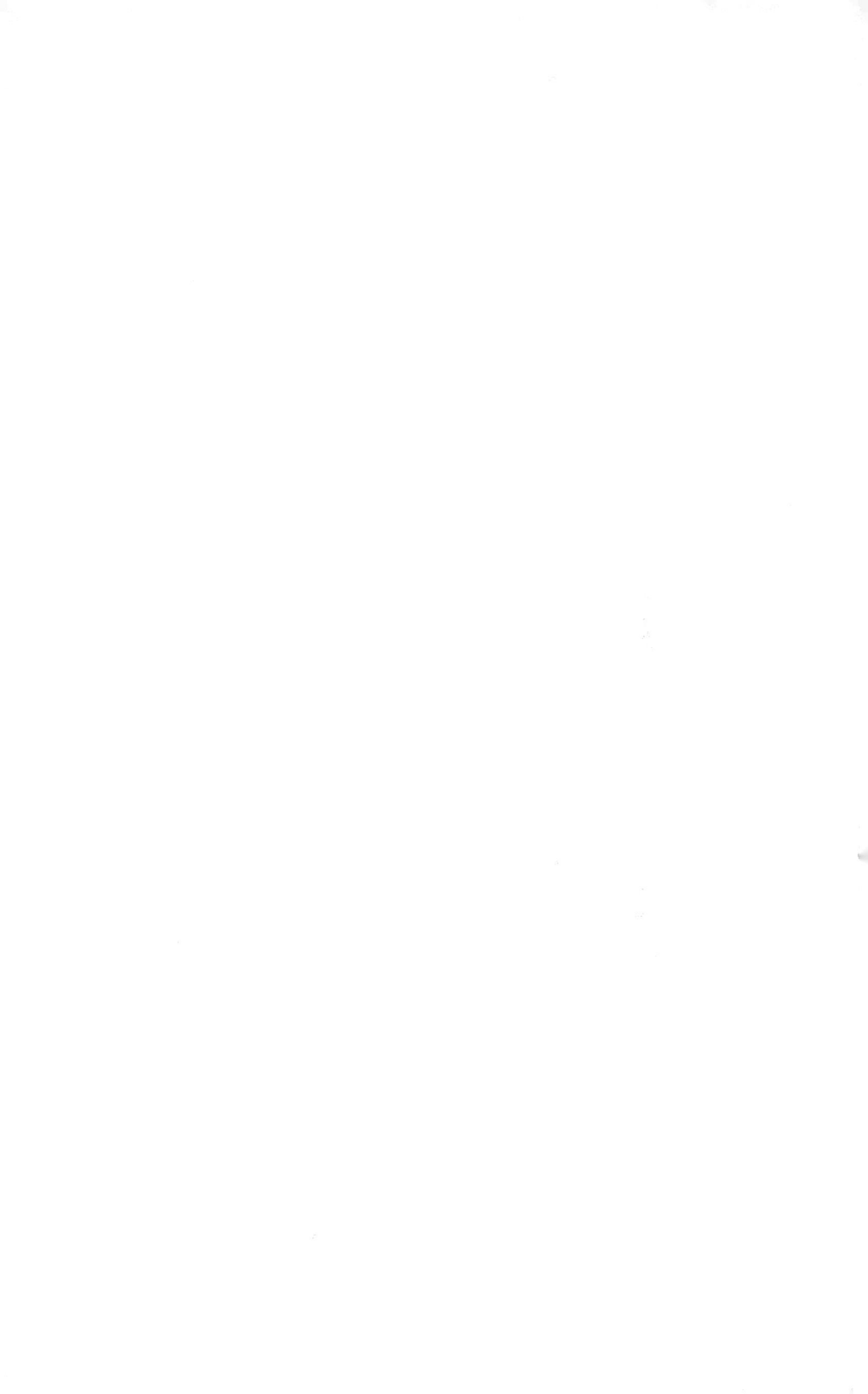

Made in the USA
Columbia, SC
03 November 2019